Gemmotherapy

Gemmotherapy

The Science of Healing with Plant Stem Cells

Roger Halfon, M.D.

Translated by Jon E. Graham

Healing Arts Press
Rochester, Vermont • Toronto, Canada

Healing Arts Press
One Park Street
Rochester, Vermont 05767
www.HealingArtsPress.com

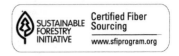

Healing Arts Press is a division of Inner Traditions International

Originally published in French under the title *La gemmothérapie ou l'embryothérapie végétale: La santé par les bourgeons* by Éditions Trajectoire
First U.S. edition published in 2010 by Healing Arts Press

Note to the reader: *This book is intended as an informational guide. The remedies, approaches, and techniques described herein are meant to supplement, and not to be a substitute for, professional medical care or treatment. They should not be used to treat a serious ailment without prior consultation with a qualified health care professional.*

Library of Congress Cataloging-in-Publication Data

Halfon, Roger.
   [Gemmothérapie, ou. L'embryothérapie végétale. English]
   Gemmotherapy : the science of healing with plant stem cells / Roger Halfon ; translated by Jon E. Graham.
      p. cm.
   Includes index.
   Originally published in French under the title: La gemmothérapie, ou, L'embryothérapie végétale. Paris : Éditions Trajectoire, c2005
   Summary: "Harnessing the vital energy of plant buds for detoxification and rejuvenation"—Provided by publisher.
   ISBN 978-1-59477-341-9 (pbk.)
   1. Buds—Therapeutic use. I. Title.
   RS164.H1813 2005
   615'.321—dc22

                                                                    2010016300

Printed and bound in the United States by Lake Book Manufacturing
The text paper is 100% SFI certified. The Sustainable Forestry Initiative˙ program promotes sustainable forest management.

10 9 8 7 6 5 4 3 2 1

Text design by Virginia L. Scott Bowman and layout by Priscilla Baker
This book was typeset in Garamond Premier Pro with Bell Gothic and Agenda used as display typefaces

Contents

Acknowledgments

I would like to pay homage to the remarkable research performed in the development of this therapy by Dr. Pol Henry, who first researched gemmotherapy; Drs. Max and Jean-Manuel Tetau, David Scimeca, and Joseph d'Esgor; and Philippe Andrianne, whose books, written in French, are essential for a comprehensive understanding of this modality.

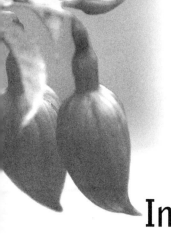

Introduction

We are living in a period of radical evolutionary change amid a succession of new technological discoveries in electronics, chemistry, and biology. Medicine has participated fully in this trend and numerous therapies have made tremendous strides, especially in the holistic field. The widespread interest in returning to nature over the last decades has reawakened older therapies that had been somewhat neglected in the face of enormous progress by medical science in the twentieth century. Their resurgence does not, however, suggest that pharmaceutical advances should be abandoned.

The use of plants for healing purposes—phytotherapy—has played a significant role in these recent developments in human health care, as it has since the dawn of time. We've gradually expanded our use of the roots, stems, and flowers harvested from the plant world for use in beverages (herbal teas), ointments, supplements, baths, and so on.

However, as we move further into the twenty-first century, many proponents of conventional medicine still decry plant-based healing as a dusty teaching that can offer nothing for the future and should be consigned to oblivion. Our modern world demands products that can be administered in precise and verifiable dosages, which traditional phytotherapy, despite its many benefits, cannot offer.

It is this dilemma that has motivated many researchers, such as

Dr. Pol Henry of Belgium (1918–1988). Extrapolating from Swiss physician Paul Niehans's controversial pioneering work in animal cell therapy of the 1930s, in 1947 Dr. Henry became particularly interested in the use of extracts made from embryonic plant matter (buds and young shoots).

Niehans had successfully used intramuscular injections of cellular crush obtained from animal embryos to stimulate human vital potential. In part because it requires a complex protocol, as well as the availability of strictly monitored livestock, this therapy is not yet universally accepted. It is, however, practiced in certain American and Swiss health establishments, where injections of embryonic cells and organs (embryo therapy) have reputedly been an excellent therapy for retriggering the immune system and initiating what could be called a rejuvenation process, particularly after the body has been purged by a draining therapy.

Henry based his work on the same principle Niehans had followed: that embryos (in this case, plant buds) contain all the cells needed for new growth (leaves, branches, and buds), as well as all of the active ingredients necessary to produce a mature entity. He called his work phytoembryotherapy.

French physician Max Tetau expanded on Pol Henry's research, and because plant buds physically resemble precious stones (*gemma,* in Latin), he described the emerging body of knowledge and healing modality as gemmotherapy. It was further developed using rigid biological methods by two medical doctors, O. A. Julian and Flament, among others.

Plant embryo therapy, also called plant stem cell therapy, or gemmotherapy—the use of buds and young plant shoots—offers the same therapeutic possibilities as animal embryo therapy and various pharmaceutical formulations, but without any side effects. Since it involves no injections, there is no possibility for rejection, shock, or even infection. The preparations are simply ingested orally or applied cutaneously.

The oral ingestion of these preparations, moreover, reveals other activities and potential of the plants, thereby contributing to a better understanding of plant-based medicine. Plant-based remedies are now being used in ways previously not even imagined.

This should not be taken as a rejection of the phytotherapy data we've already gleaned from such healing agents as herbal teas, aromatherapy, Bach Flower Remedies, and so on. This new understanding both emphasizes the effectiveness of plant use in familiar modalities and supports the discovery of new applications and therapies.

The fig tree, for example, traditionally has been used only for its laxative properties, but gemmotherapy research has revealed that its buds have an effect on the cortico-hypothalamic axis. This makes them anxiolytic (anti-anxiety) agents that could be very useful in the treatment of all psychosomatic disorders.

Black currant may be better known to many people as cassis, a French aperitif made famous by a priest of Dijon, France. Felix Kir was formerly mayor of that city and a hero of the French Resistance during World War II, but today he is best remembered for the dry white wine and cassis aperitif that bears his name. Had Kir been aware that the buds of this rambling, thorny plant possess a powerful anti-inflammatory action that rivals that of cortisone, he might instead be remembered as a hero of natural healing.

Gemmotherapy extracts are also useful for cleansing our bodies from troublesome or even dangerous chemicals. This detoxification at the cellular level can remove toxins that might otherwise prevent replication of healthy cells, thereby causing disease and organ failure.

As these examples demonstrate, gemmotherapy is at the heart of a brand-new field of natural therapy with major potential for both its indications and its applications. Although the list of remedies presented here is not exhaustive, it includes thirty-four of the most common gemmotherapy extracts currently in use.

The purpose of this book is to introduce and explain this subject in such a way that everyone may benefit, but as with all active therapies, gemmotherapy should be practiced only under the supervision and guidance of a trained health professional.

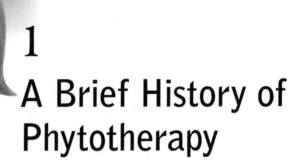

1
A Brief History of Phytotherapy

Gemmotherapy is the newest therapy to come to light in the field of plant medicine. Plant-based medicine, or phytotherapy, is one of humanity's oldest healing practices.

It is highly likely that phytotherapy was first practiced by our earliest human ancestors, who instinctively would have turned to the environment nearest their caves in search of treatments for their various ailments. The oldest known written record of healing plants is on Sumerian clay tablets that date back as early as 2100 BCE.

Legend tells us that Aristotle persuaded Alexander the Great to use certain plants in treating his soldiers' wounds in the fourth century BCE, and the Chinese also studied botany in that time period. By 60 CE a Greek physician named Dioscorides had produced *De Materia Medica,* which described more than a thousand medicines, about 60 percent of which were plant based. In that same era, Pliny, a Roman who perished in the eruption of Mt. Vesuvius, wrote his monumental *Historia Naturalis,* which included vast sections on medicinal herbs.

Plants have been used in countless ways throughout history and some species have played a critical role in human development. For example, the discovery of the New World was triggered by the desire for spices, and discovery ships of that era often included either a botanist who supervised collection of new species samples to bring back to Europe for study and cultivation, or an artist who drew renderings of new species for identification by botanists in the home country.

Tobacco and chocolate were both introduced into the French court as medicinal plants after they'd been discovered in the new world. Catherine de Medici smoked "Nicot's herb" to relieve her migraines, and Louis XV treated his "fatigue" with a cup of chocolate.

Herbal knowledge spread from France throughout the courts of Europe over the sixteenth and seventeenth centuries. Eventually its "letter of nobility" was the creation of a diploma for those who excelled in its study. However, the twentieth century saw this academic honor suspended by a decree of the Vichy government on September 11, 1941: "Diplomas in herbalism will no longer be issued and only those who already have such a diploma may continue to practice this profession." This was a huge setback for plant healing, and invalidated (at least in France) more than two thousand years of study and contemplation.

HISTORICAL HIGHLIGHTS OF PLANT MEDICINE

If we trace the recorded history of this science back to its earliest known origins, we see that it was practiced throughout the known world. The ancient Egyptians appear to have acquired a great mastery of this field. One of their significant accomplishments was the embalming of bodies, which they raised to a high art.

A Chinese document that formed the basis of traditional Chinese medicine (TCM) is actually two books known collectively as the *Yellow Emperor's Classic of Internal Medicine*. Some experts believe the first book was written over the course of several centuries, from the third century BCE to 1053 CE, but it is the second book that offers details on the properties of certain plants, and on which TCM is based.

In India, the *Atharva Veda,* one of the Vedic texts that date as far back as the second millennium BCE, describes various maladies and their herbal remedies. Another Vedic text, the *Caraka Samhita,* is considered to be the authoritative treatise on ayurveda and includes 341 recipes made from plants.

Hippocrates (460–377 BCE), known as the father of modern medicine, stressed the use of rosemary and garlic in healing, and attempted to clarify which herbs were efficacious.

The Persian doctor Avicenna (981–1037 CE) emphasized the use of plants in his tome: *The Canon of Medicine.*

A Swiss citizen who adopted the Latin name Paracelsus developed his *Doctrine of Signatures* in sixteenth-century Europe. This doctrine connects the physical appearance of a plant with the human organ it most resembles: "What resembles the organ treats the organ." An active proponent of treating with plants, Paracelsus believed that plants with yellow sap were cures for jaundice, long-lived plants were used to attempt to lengthen life, and ailments of the lower part of the body were treated with below-ground plant parts.

In seventeenth-century England, the doctor and astrologer Nicholas Culpeper translated the Latin text *Pharmacopoeia* into his native tongue. This text listed the qualities of a number of plants and allowed him to spread the science of phytotherapy to his medical colleagues.

In nineteenth-century America, Samuel Thompson wrote a number of treatises concerning what he had learned about Native American healing traditions. His disciple, Dr. Coffin, was driven from the United States by the jealousy of a professional colleague and moved to the northern part of England in 1864, where he created the National Association of Practicing Herbalists. Coffin's work undoubtedly had an influence on Dr. Edward Bach, who created the Bach Flower Remedies at the beginning of the twentieth century. These are still widely used today.

Plant medicine recovered from the Vichy ban and enjoyed a period of renewal in France in the 1950s, spearheaded by Maurice Messegue, Jean Valnet, and Michel Bontemps. Their work triggered a renewed and keen interest in this body of knowledge. This was also the time during which gemmotherapy was born from the work and studies of Pol Henry, Max Tetau, and their colleagues.

PHYTOTHERAPY PREPARATIONS

Historically, gemmotherapy belongs to the body of knowledge known as phytotherapy, or plant medicine traditions. There are unique laws and forms used in plant-based medical treatments.

Two principles have always been applied in all medical traditions that are based on the use of herbs and other plants:

1. The wild plant is always preferable to the one grown domestically, because its best environment and climate are those provided by nature, thus the active elements they contain are at their strongest when growing in the wild.
2. It's best to select the plants that have the strongest aroma, deepest color, and thickest buds (perhaps an early manifestation of the idea of gemmotherapy).

The earliest known phytotherapy preparations were water-based, as water provided the simplest and most effective means for extracting the constituent elements of plants. These preparations included infusions (herbal teas), baths, herb macerations, and marinations for tinctures.

Infusions

An herbal tea is a beverage that contains a low dose of an infused plant substance with medicinal properties. It is prepared by placing a handful of fresh or dried herbs in a container and pouring very hot water (not boiling, which can alter the herb's properties) over it. This water should also be as pure as possible.

The herbs are left to steep in this water for three to eight minutes, depending on the density and part of the plant used. Flowers require less time than roots and stems. The resulting infusion is consumed at a lukewarm temperature, sweetened to preference. An average of one to six cups may be drunk every day, depending on the individual's needs.

Decoctions

Decoctions are called for when using bark, some roots, or very tough seeds. Their action is often much stronger than that of teas or infusions.

To prepare a decoction, the plant matter is placed in cold water and brought to a boil for about fifteen minutes, which reduces the liquid to a thicker fluid. Decoctions are also used in preparing syrups, which are simply decoctions to which sugar or honey has been added. The Romans created healing ointments by adding a grated apple and lard to herbal decoctions.

Macerations

Macerations are made by placing a specific quantity of plant matter in liquid and allowing it to steep for a time period that can range anywhere from several hours to several weeks. Homeopathy uses maceration to extract the plant properties used as mother tinctures from which homeopathic dilutions are prepared.

Water is not the ideal liquid for making macerations because it can lead to fermentation over the extended time period. People in ancient times turned to wine and alcohol, knowing that red wine possesses astringent qualities due to its high tannin content, and that white wine has a tendency to be diuretic.

Much later, at the beginning of the twentieth century, the English doctor Bach used brandy and cognac in the preparation of his wild flower elixirs.

Creams and Ointments

Oil and fat were added to certain plants or their macerations to make oils, creams, ointments, and pomades (a blend of oil and alcohol applied directly to the skin).

Therapeutic Immersion

Baths have been available since ancient times, whether for hygiene or healing. Some cultures used mineral water scented with aromatic plants.

Early Romans bathed daily at the *caldarium,* often following their cleansing with a massage. On the other side of the world, the Japanese culture has a long history of bathing for both hygiene and pleasure.

Throughout the ages, baths have been a social ritual as much as a hygienic endeavor. In the Middle Ages it was not infrequent to have banquets at the baths, with feasts served on floating tables and a musician seated in the water along with the guests.

In Paris in the year 1300 there were twenty-five public baths where herbal therapies were also available. These same treatments can be found today in spas specializing in thalassotherapy, a natural healing treatment that uses seawater to increase circulation and restore depleted minerals.

The Catholic clergy cast a dim eye on men and women bathing together, and banned all baths in which men and women shared the same tubs around 1400.

In the sixteenth and seventeenth centuries, baths experienced greatly diminished popularity due to concerns that the water was spreading disease, but in the eighteenth century, when it became obvious that the opposite was true, bathing came back into favor. In fact, some of the nobility, both gentlemen and ladies, would even receive visitors while immersed in baths enhanced with decoctions of numerous aromatic plants.

Among the plants most popular for baths were thyme, sage, marjoram, and rosemary for their tonic properties; and lavender, cypress, and pine for their circulatory and antispasmodic qualities.

Capsules

In the second half of the twentieth century there was increasing use of plant concentrates in capsules, a form with ease of ingestion that is perfectly adapted to the needs of the modern world. However, something was lost in the process, because plants that have been dried and powdered have also been stripped of a substantial amount of their active qualities. This brings us back to the use of buds and embryonic plant tissue, which now appears to be the most active and promising form of plant medicine.

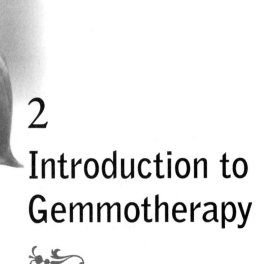

2
Introduction to Gemmotherapy

As noted earlier, gemmotherapy uses plant buds and other living embryonic tissue (shoots and radicels, which are small roots or rootlets branching off from the main root) for deep drainage of the body and to regularize the function of distressed organs. It uses the high concentration of growth factors in these embryonic plant tissues to effect these results through the nervous system and the reticuloendothelial system (RES).

In this book we are concentrating on the most available gemmotherapy extracts, preparations based on thirty-four different plants, but ongoing research is likely to expand this number.

The extracts are prepared from fresh buds or young plant shoot tissues, which are chopped and left to macerate in a blend of water, glycerin, and alcohol. This particular solution appears to be the best solvent and support material for the properties of the plants.

After they have been steeped for three weeks, which is the length of time that tests indicate is required for the active qualities in this tissue to be fully released, the brew is pressed and filtered. The resulting product is the full-strength concentrated extract, currently not sold in U.S. retail stores but available to doctors who can order the remedies for their patients.

MOST COMMON PLANTS CURRENTLY USED IN GEMMOTHERAPY

Alder	*Alnus glutinosa*
Ash	*Fraxinus excelsior*
Birch	*Betula pendula*
Black currant	*Ribes nigrum*
Bloodtwig dogwood	*Cornus sanguinea*
Bramble or blackberry	*Rubus fructicosus*
Cedar of Lebanon	*Cedrus libanus*
Chestnut	*Castanea sativa*
English walnut	*Juglans regia*
Field elm	*Ulmus minor*
Fig tree	*Ficus carica*
Grapevine	*Vitis vinifera*
Hawthorn	*Crataegus oxyacantha*
Hazel	*Corylus avellana*
Heather	*Calluna vulgaris*
Hedge maple	*Acer campestre*
Hornbeam	*Carpinus betulus*
Horse chestnut	*Aesculus hippocastanum*
Juniper	*Juniperus communis*
Lemon tree	*Citrus limonum*
Lilac	*Syringa vulgaris*
Lingonberry	*Vaccinium vitis idaea*
Oak	*Quercus robur*
Olive tree	*Olea europaea*
Raspberry bush	*Rubus idaeus*
Rosemary	*Rosmarinus officinalis*
Rowan	*Sorbus domestica*
Scots pine	*Pinus sylvestris*
Sequoia	*Sequoia gigantea*
Silver linden	*Tilia tomentosa*
Tamarind	*Tamarix gallica*
Wayfaring tree	*Viburnum lantana*
White willow	*Salix alba*
Wild or dog rose	*Rosa canina*

The maceration can then be diluted ten times and dynamized homeopathically to create a dilution of the first decimal, known as D1 (or 1X). This fluid should be one twentieth of the weight of the plant tissue that was initially collected. The D1 homeopathic strength remedies are available in retail markets (see Resources for further information).

Both the homeopathic D1 dilution and the macerated concentrate are most frequently taken orally in the form of drops, but can also be taken as a spray or applied in a cream. Since the effects are powerful, it's best to secure the guidance of a health professional to help you determine the appropriate product and dosage.

In general, the following dosages are recommended:

D1 homeopathic strength: 50 to 100 drops in water two times daily

Full-strength concentrated extract: 5 to 15 drops twice daily, taken in a little water

Oral spray: D1 maceration can also be used as an oral spray. In this case the treatment consists of applying the spray to the mucous membranes of the tongue one to three times a day.

These different forms are all effective and their selection is generally based on practicality and availability. The powerful life force in the initial buds and young shoots will be present in any event. All contain the entire genetic material held in the plant, which contains many highly concentrated growth factors (gibberellins) that will stimulate the body's vital potential and regenerative capacities. This, in turn, will make it possible for the body to recover its natural ability to eliminate toxins and fulfill its physiological functions at an optimum level.

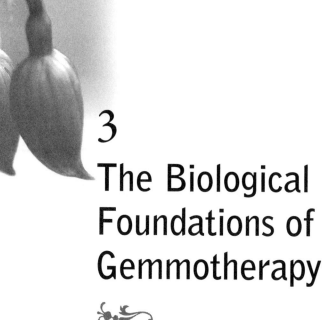

3

The Biological Foundations of Gemmotherapy

Once they had established a basis for this new therapy, Pol Henry and Max Tetau focused their attention on more extensively analyzing the biological data unearthed by their initial studies. Their research focused on three principal core areas, as follows:

CHEMICAL ANALYSIS

Buds and young shoots were chemically analyzed to determine how their constituent elements differed from the adult plants.

By using chromatography on extremely thin layers, the doctors were able to uncover evidence of a much higher level of active properties in buds than in fully grown plants. For example, black currant (*Ribes nigrum*) buds revealed four times more antioxidizing pycnogenols than were found in preparations made from fully developed leaves. Tests also revealed that the level of amino acids was 40 percent higher, and that some amino acids gradually disappeared entirely in the leaf stage.

Black currant bud also contains a substantial quantity of vitamin C (17 mg/g), which is twice as much as that found in the adult plant.

ISOLATED MOLECULE VERSUS ENTIRE PLANT

Researchers investigated the pharmacological properties of the isolated molecule in comparison with an isolated active property of the entire plant.

This study used a variety of tests, such as the Halpern test (see below) to show evidence of the product's activity on the level of the reticuloendothelial system (RES), which is part of the immune system. Reticuloendothelial cells are phagocytic, meaning they can ingest or destroy viruses and other foreign substances, as well as abnormal body cells.

The Halpern test is based on the fact that the RES collects so-called vital colors in its cells, such as trypan blue and lithium carmine. This makes it possible to assess the collecting power of the macerated particles when they are injected intravenously in various parts of the reticuloendothelial system.

The research started with tests using birch on two groups of albino rats. One group was given a gemmotherapy extract made from birch buds for ten days, and the other was given a simple extract from the leaves. Test results revealed a very significant stimulation of the immune system in the rats fed the birch gemmotherapy extract, a much stronger response than was seen in those given the leaf extract.

Further tests were then successfully conducted using silver linden (also known as lime tree or white lime) to study the nervous system, hawthorn for analyzing the cardiovascular effects of these extracts, and rosemary for testing their hepatic (impact on the liver) effects.

All of these tests provided positive results for the gemmotherapy macerated extracts.

COMPARATIVE CLINICAL STUDIES

Following the other tests, comparative clinical studies were performed on three patient test groups: a group receiving the macerated gemmotherapy extract, another receiving an extract produced from the entire plant, and a third group receiving a placebo containing nothing but distilled water.

Results of these tests clearly demonstrated the superior action of gemmotherapy extracts over basic preparations, and made it possible to identify their core therapeutic action.

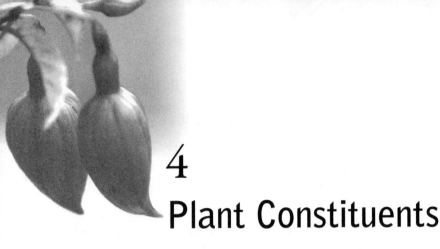

4
Plant Constituents

Every plant is a conglomeration of numerous elements, and it is most likely that each plant owes its properties and unique identity to the way all these molecules are combined and work together.

Before introducing the primary thirty-four most common plants currently being macerated to produce gemmotherapy extracts, it might be helpful to have a quick general review of what chemical analysis reveals about a plant. Plants are composed of the following constituent elements:

- *Alkaloids,* the action of which is variable (and sometimes toxic), but from which we derive such important substances as caffeine, morphine, and nicotine.
- *Anthraquinones,* substances that generally have a laxative and fat-eliminating effect upon the body.
- *Betulin,* which has antiviral and anti-inflammatory properties.
- *Coumarins,* which are a precursor of some anticoagulants.
- *Ericodine,* which is a highly antiseptic and diuretic alkaloid.
- *Flavonoids,* known for their antioxidant activity and effect on the blood vessels and circulatory level. They also have diuretic properties.
- *Gamma-linolenic acid,* which is an essential omega-6 fatty acid.

- *Glucosides,* which are very similar to glucose and can often have a calming effect upon the heart and lungs.
- *Juglones,* which have fungicidal and antibiotic properties.
- *Lignans,* which are estrogen-like chemicals that act as antioxidants and are a building block for cell walls.
- *Linoleic acid,* which is an essential omega-6 fatty acid.
- *Mucilages* and *gums,* which are endowed with soothing qualities and help the scarring process.
- *Napthoquinones,* which possess a laxative action similar to that of anthraquinones.
- *Saponins,* substances that, on contact with water, have an emulsifying effect that softens skin.
- *Tannins,* anti-inflammatory and antiseptic molecules that create the astringent quality of some preparations.
- *Terpenes,* which in plants are typically found as a component of the plant's essential oils.
- *Vitamins* and *trace elements* can also be discovered in some plants.

All of these elements appear in a concentrated form in the buds, young shoots, and rootlets of plants.

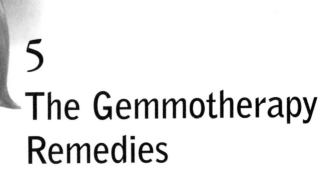

5
The Gemmotherapy Remedies

Materia Medica

This chapter, covering thirty-four common gemmotherapy preparations, is presented in alphabetical order, with each plant's common name followed by its Latin botanical name. An overview of the principal actions of each of the remedies is included at the beginning for easy reference. The use and dosage of the gemmotherapy remedies presented here should be based on an individual's diagnosis and professional recommendations of a doctor or other health professional. (General dosage guidelines were provided in chapter 2; see also chapter 6.)

OVERVIEW: PRINCIPAL ACTIONS OF GEMMOTHERAPY REMEDIES

Gemmotherapy Remedy	Principal Action
Alder	Facilitates cerebral circulation
Ash	Supports the osteoarticular system, restores body's mineral content
Birch	Purifier (triggers diuresis), helps rheumatism and skin problems
Black currant	Antiallergenic

Gemmotherapy Remedy	Principal Action
Bloodtwig dogwood	Helps prevent coronaries, heart attacks
Bramble or Blackberry	Useful for bronchitis, emphysema; strengthens bones
Cedar of Lebanon	Drains skin of impurities
Chestnut	Tonic, acts on lymphatic system
English walnut	Supports intestines and skin
Field elm	Drains skin of impurities
Fig tree	Aids all psychosomatic disorders, especially those affecting the stomach
Grapevine	Aids chronic inflammations, osteoarticular system, prostate
Hazel	Acts on lungs (emphysema and asthma)
Hawthorn	Supports heart and healthy blood pressure
Heather	Acts on urinary system
Hedge maple	Helpful for digestion, gallbladder
Hornbeam	Acts on blood (platelets, edemas, varicose ulcers)
Horse chestnut	Helpful for vein circulation, hemorrhoids
Juniper	Liver drainer
Lemon tree	Blood thinner, helps arteritis and varicose veins
Lilac	Supports cardiovascular system, antirheumatic
Lingonberry	Good for intestines
Oak	Tonic
Olive tree	Acts on cerebral circulation
Raspberry bush	Supports female hormonal system (ovaries)
Rosemary	Liver remedy, tonic
Rowan	Acts on veins
Scots pine	Acts on osteoarticular system, restores mineral content to body
Sequoia	Hormonal tonic (primarily for men)
Silver linden	Autonomic tranquilizer
Tamarind	Stimulates red blood cells and coagulation
Wayfaring tree	Pulmonary action
White willow	Analgesic, anti-inflammatory
Wild or dog rose	Supports ear, nose, and throat

🌿 Alder

Alnus glutinosa

The alder tree is fond of water and humidity, which is one reason why it is most commonly found on the banks of small streams and rivers, as well as on adjacent flood plains. Alder fruits strongly resemble small pinecones.

Plant Constituents

Alder, a tree recognizable by its dentate leaves (the edges resemble teeth), contains lignans, 20 percent tannin, and glucosides.

Traditional Uses

Alder wood, with its property of hardening when immersed in water, was the primary building material used for constructing the Italian city of Venice. It was also in this city that decoctions of alder bark were recommended for blood purification, beverages, and mouthwashes that are still efficacious today.

A mouthwash can be made by boiling a half ounce of the bark in a half pint of water, letting it cool to lukewarm, and gargling with it several times a day. The bark's astringent properties help to alleviate inflammation and tighten mucous membranes.

These astringent properties were taken advantage of in Spain, where pilgrims applied alder leaves to their weary, aching feet.

Alder has also been used to alleviate rheumatism, mastitis, and some skin infections.

The Gemmotherapy Remedy

The part of the plant used to make the gemmotherapy remedy is the bud.

Principal Action

Alder acts essentially on problems with blood circulation, most particularly cases of arteritis (inflammation of artery walls) and phlebitis (vein inflammation).

It also improves cerebral circulation, which makes it highly valuable for treating strokes and problems of senility and memory loss, and it is extremely helpful in the treatment of migraines.

Secondary Action

This gemmotherapy extract shows evidence of being useful in combating allergies, and thus can be recommended for the treatment of hives and all other allergy symptoms. It also has antispasmodic effects on the colon and stomach.

Dosage

The general dosage guidelines are in accordance with those previously mentioned (see page 12). However, in the case of migraines, sufferers should use one spraying, or 5 drops, once an hour.

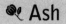

Ash

Fraxinus excelsior

Ash is a deciduous tree with a light-colored bark. Its silvery gray color, black buds, and flowers without petals all make it easily recognizable. Its wood is quite flexible and supple, and could almost be described as elastic.

Plant Constituents

The leaves of the ash tree contain flavonoids, tannins, terpenes, and mucilages.

Traditional Uses

Ash is known as the "tree of life" in Norse mythology, with roots that stretch down into the world of the gods and branches that spread wide into infinity.

According to Celtic tradition, the first man was carved from this tree, and as a testament to ash's invigorating qualities, it was customary in Scotland prior to the nineteenth century to give newborns a spoonful of ash sap to strengthen and fortify them. Its bark was also commonly used for treating fever before the cinchona (from which quinine is produced) was discovered.

The Gemmotherapy Remedy

The part used to manufacture this extract is the bud of the leaf.

Principal Action

This particular gemmotherapy extract reveals properties of the ash tree that were scarcely known before. For example, ash in this instance acts specifically on the joints—perhaps because of this tree's singular flexibility, if we accept the medical doctrine of signatures postulated by

Paracelsus. It can also be considered one of the preeminent remedies for treating rheumatism.

Secondary Action

In connection with its powerful action against rheumatism, ash also has a strong purgative and laxative effect that greatly contributes to purifying the bloodstream.

❧ Birch (Silver Birch)

Betula pendula

The silver birch tree often grows to a height of ninety feet. Its slender, scaly trunk is covered by a pale gray or white bark that strongly resembles paper. Its name may be even be derived from the Sanskrit word *bharga,* which means "writing support."

This tree can be found throughout Europe and North America, predominantly in northern areas, and it is in these same northern regions that it has been most often used for its healing properties.

Plant Constituents

The most active part of this tree is its essential oil, which contains methyl salicylate. Betulin can be found in the bark of this tree.

Traditional Uses

The silver birch is a tree of universal potential, originally used primarily in the northern countries of Europe. It was used to make wooden shoes, brooms, and rope, and its sap was used as a substitute for sugar in the preparation of wine.

In Russia, an oil extracted from this tree was used to perfume leather and mask its animal scent. In the kitchen it was used for brewing beer and for a purée that some indigenous Russian peoples mixed with caviar. Its dried leaves were brewed in a tea intended to prevent weight gain and were also used as a tobacco substitute.

In fact, birch is the preeminent purifying tree, a quality that inspired Italian medical doctor and botanist Mathiole to write in 1565: "If the trunk of the birch is pierced with an auger, it will release a large quantity of sap that has a powerful property and virtue for breaking down kidney and bladder stones if used continuously. This fluid removes patches from the face and makes the skin plump and beautiful. If you wash your mouth with it, it will heal any mouth ulcers present inside."

In the nineteenth century, surgeon Pierre-François Percy noted:

"Throughout northern Europe, starting from our own regions by the Rhine to the northernmost reaches of Russia, birch water is the hope, happiness, and panacea of all inhabitants rich and poor, large and small, lords and serfs. Skin disorders like acne, scurf patches, and broken veins are rarely able to resist its power. It is a valuable remedy against all rheumatic disorders, the remnants of gout, and bladder problems, as well as for a host of chronic ills against which medical science is prone to fail."

The Gemmotherapy Remedy

The parts of the plant used to make the gemmotherapy remedy are the buds and rootlets, both of which amplify its traditionally ascribed healing properties.

Principal Action

Because of its powerful purifying properties and its activation of diuresis and uric acid elimination, birch has proven itself to be an essential remedy for the treatment of rheumatism, kidney disorders, and skin problems.

Secondary Action

There is a new therapeutic property revealed by gemmotherapy birch extract. The macerated birch bud has demonstrated that it is also a strong stimulant of the endocrine system, and because of its effect on the corticoadrenal glands, it has the potential to address certain sexual disorders, such as impotence and frigidity. This property also makes it useful for combating certain depressive states.

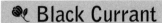 Black Currant

Ribes nigrum

The original native regions for black currant appear to be the Himalayas and the plains of Nepal. It is a bush that grows to an average of four or five feet tall and produces black berries with a bittersweet flavor.

Plant Constituents

The berries contain a high level of vitamin C, sugars, and flavonoids, which are useful for addressing circulatory problems.

Black currant seeds, however, contain linoleic acids and 18 percent gamma-linolenic acid, which makes this bush a very important tool for health professionals.

Traditional Uses

In ancient times, black currant leaves reputedly had the ability to heal cuts and wounds made by blades and other sharp instruments. The leaves were known to be effective against inflammation caused by bee stings, and for treating whitlow—a painful viral infection in one or more fingers (now known to be caused primarily by herpes simplex)—and gout. Finally, black currant was also recommended as an appetite stimulant.

Black currant was referred to as the "good savior." Hildegard von Bingen recommended it as a panacea, and in 1712 it was dubbed the Elixir of Life by P. Bailly, the abbot of Montaran, because of its positive effect on longevity: "Black currant maintains health so well that it often makes the elderly appear much younger than they truly are."

The Gemmotherapy Remedy

The part of the plant used to make the gemmotherapy remedy is the bud.

Principal Action

If you had to choose only one gemmotherapy extract to take with you to a desert island, it would have to be black currant. It has high vitamin C content and is a powerful immune system booster.

Black currant has a powerful stimulating effect on the adrenal glands, and has proven to be one of the preeminent antiallergenic and anti-inflammatory agents available. It is as powerful as cortisone without any of the adverse side effects.

It is an indispensable remedy for the treatment of osteoarthritis and other painful joint disorders, as well as one for treating various skin allergies, such as psoriasis and eczema.

Secondary Action

Thanks to its constituent elements, black currant provides an excellent remedy against fatigue, including both physical and mental exhaustion. It is also highly effective against all kinds of infections.

Bloodtwig Dogwood

Cornus sanguinea

A native plant of Japan, China, and Korea, bloodtwig dogwood (also known as "midwinter fire") is a deciduous tree with shiny leaves and oval red berries. It was mentioned in the earliest Chinese herbals as one of the ingredients in the "wonderful eight element pill." The other seven ingredients were pepper, salt, honey, seaweed, swallows' nest, mare's milk, and tea leaves.

Plant Constituents

Bloodtwig dogwood contains glucosides, saponins, and tannins.

Traditional Uses

This tree was used by the ancient Romans and Chinese to reduce abnormally high fluid secretions from the body, such as overly frequent urination or heavy perspiration.

The Gemmotherapy Remedy

The part of the plant used to make the gemmotherapy remedy is the bud.

Principal Action

The gemmotherapy extract formulated with the macerated buds of this tree has a powerful effect on the heart and bloodstream. For example, bloodtwig dogwood "washes" clogged arteries clean, hence its indication for use in the treatment of arteritis. More importantly, bloodtwig dogwood exhibits properties that are helpful in supporting arteries to combat arteriosclerosis.

This tree's extract also has a positive effect on blood fluidity, which makes it an important therapeutic adjunct for treating heart failure and protecting against heart attack.

Also, because it stimulates circulation in the veins, bloodtwig dogwood can be recommended against the cold feet disorder that affects a large number of people during the winter.

Secondary Action

Bloodtwig dogwood buds also have an effect on the thyroid, regulating thyroid function by either stimulating or slowing it. Stimulation of the thyroid also contributes to increased body temperature and metabolism, which may explain its anti-chill effect on the body's extremities.

❧ Bramble or Blackberry

Rubus fruticosus

The blackberry is a low-growing, rambling, extremely hardy and invasive perennial commonly found in hedgerows, wastelands, ditches, vacant lots, wooded areas, and uncultivated areas all over the temperate zones of the Northern Hemisphere.

Its long, reddish, arching stems are equipped with tough curved thorns that lacerate the hands of anyone who gets too close.

The rough leaves of this plant grow in an alternating pattern and consist of three to five oval folioles and a prickly petiole. The leaves are dark green on top, and the underside is downy-white.

The pink or white flowers are arranged in terminal clusters and flower in the period from June to August.

The fruit from which this shrub gets one of its names, blackberry, is comprised of numerous drupelets that turn black or deep purple as they ripen. The fruit is harvested in September.

Plant Constituents

Blackberry bushes are rich in tannins, sugars, and gums; and malic, succininc, and citric acids.

Traditional Uses

The Latin name for this plant, *rubus* (from which its French name, *ronce,* is derived), means dart, in reference to its hooked thorns that can easily snag clothing and scratch unwary body parts. Long before they began to be regarded as a gourmet autumnal treat, unripened blackberries were often used for health purposes.

Theophrastus and Dioscorides were fully aware of the plant's astringent virtues, and Hildegard von Bingen praised its qualities for treating coughs, sore throats, and toothaches. She also demonstrated that when its fresh leaves were crushed between the fingers and rubbed over the skin, bleeding would immediately stop. This explains why it is often prescribed for bleeding hemorrhoids or unusually heavy menstrual flow.

The blackberry bush's life force is so strong that the plant can be cultivated inside a test tube. If a small piece of a blackberry stem is placed on a nutritive base of agar in the tube and given regular care, in several months a blackberry bush shoot will begin to grow there.

The Gemmotherapy Remedy

The part of the plant used to make the gemmotherapy remedy is the young shoot.

Principal Action

Macerated blackberry reveals anti-fibrous properties that are effective in addressing pulmonary issues. This makes it an effective weapon against emphysema and episodes of chronic bronchitis.

Macerated blackberry undeniably provides flexibility to the pulmonary alveoli, thus contributing to the expansion of respiratory capacity.

Secondary Action

Blackberry also greatly helps to restore the body's necessary mineral content, which makes it highly beneficial in treating a fracture. The bone's ability to fuse and repair will be helped immensely.

& Cedar of Lebanon

Cedrus libanus

The cedar is one of the tallest and most majestic of all trees. It can grow as high as 140 feet (and heights of 200 feet in the wild have been reported). Legend maintains that Lebanon cedar was used to build Jerusalem's Temple of Solomon and the Hanging Gardens of Babylon, because of the splendor of the wood and the qualities of its oil (also used in making incense and perfume).

Plant Constituents

Cedar contains an oil with antiseptic and diuretic properties. This cedrine oil has a very distinctive aroma and is a natural chemical for keeping away bugs.

Traditional Uses

Cedar's antiseptic and bronchial properties have been used for centuries to treat the common health afflictions of winter. In addition, a decoction made from cedar was reputedly capable of healing wounds.

The Gemmotherapy Remedy

The part of the plant used to make the gemmotherapy remedy is the bud.

Principal Action

In addition to its antiseptic and pulmonary properties, this gemmotherapy extract has revealed a new healing capacity of cedar buds. It has a significant effect on skin conditions, because the buds have a remarkable ability to trigger cutaneous draining. This is why this extract is indicated for the treatment of all skin disorders, such as eczema, psoriasis, and chronic dermatosis.

Secondary Action

In tandem with its beneficial effects on pulmonary functions, cedar macerated for gemmotherapy also soothes digestive disorders.

🌹 Chestnut (Sweet or Spanish Chestnut)

Castanea sativa

A native of the Mediterranean basin, this particular species of chestnut tree now grows throughout Europe.

Young Spanish chestnut has a smooth bark and can grow to heights of one hundred feet. The flowers from female catkins bear spiny yellow green cupules containing three to seven nuts. These cupules are also known as "burrs."

Plant Constituents

The tree contains tannins, glucides, and primarily mucilages.

Traditional Uses

In earlier times the chief uses of chestnuts were nutritional. They were roasted, made into a paste, or ground into flour. Sometimes the flowers of the chestnut tree were added to aromatic seventeenth-century tobacco blends to increase their flavor.

Teas and infusions made from chestnut trees had a reputation for healing whooping cough and other respiratory disorders.

In Bach Flower therapy, Dr. Bach recommended sweet chestnut for those who were incapable of learning from experience and were continuously making the same mistakes. Sweet Chestnut remedy enables them to refocus, analyze their real situation, and deduce its future consequences if current behavior is left unchecked.

The Gemmotherapy Remedy

The part of the plant used to make the gemmotherapy remedy is the bud.

Principal Action

Gemmotherapy reveals sweet chestnut's vital action on the lymphatic system, edemas, and vein problems, including varicose veins and hemorrhoids.

For this reason it is one of the best possible remedies for varicose ulcers, particularly when combined with cedar and black currant.

Secondary Action

Chestnut buds have an antispasmodic property that is very useful for treating colitis.

🌹 English Walnut

Juglans regia

The English walnut is actually a native of Persia that gradually migrated into Europe by way of Greece, Italy, and France. It is slow to reach maturity and takes eight years to attain its full height. The fruit of the walnut, which is surrounded by a hard shell, resembles the brain.

Plant Constituents

Walnuts contain napthoquinones, which possess a laxative action similar to that of anthraquinones, and also contain the organic compounds juglones, which have antibacterial properties.

Traditional Uses

The Latin name for the majestic walnut—*Juglans regia*—may be derived from *Jovis gland,* which means Jupiter's acorn.

Its properties and virtues have been used in various ways over the centuries. The fluid from its leaves was used for draining the liver in ancient times, and a decoction made from this tree was used for the treatment of eye problems.

Because of their shape, walnuts were used—in accordance with the doctrine of signatures (what resembles an organ can be used to treat problems suffered by that organ)—as a brain tonic.

It is interesting to note that a recipe from the Middle Ages recommended cooking the leaves and nuts of this tree in pork lard in order to make an ointment, which, when applied consistently during the time of the waxing moon, was believed to encourage the growth of hair.

The Gemmotherapy Remedy

The part of the plant used to make the gemmotherapy remedy is the bud.

The gemmotherapy extract made from walnut buds has demonstrated a powerful effect on the colon.

Principal Action

Walnut primarily targets the digestive system, especially the colon. It is recommended for treating diarrhea and helps intestinal flora reestablish itself following antibiotic treatment, which makes this extract extremely useful in the present day.

Secondary Action

The extract also demonstrates properties concerning the skin. Psoriasis, eczema, and acne have all responded favorably to treatment with walnut extract because of its purifying action that works in tandem with its intestinal action.

Walnut has also demonstrated an ability to retard the development of cataracts.

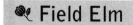 Field Elm

Ulmus minor

The elm is a majestic tree that can grow as tall as 120 feet. Its bark is cracked and it produces clusters of small red flowers that begin to appear in March. Its fruit consists of a single seed encapsulated in a *samara* (wings) that allows it to be carried by the wind.

The field elm's native range is primarily southern Europe but extends eastward into Asia Minor and as far north as the Baltics. Elms of all varieties vanished almost entirely from the European and North American continents during the 1960s and '70s because of Dutch elm disease. This affliction destroyed the tree's leaves and spread rapidly, which led to the chopping down of almost all the field elms in Europe. One distinctive feature of this species of elm is the ease with which it reproduces suckers from roots and stumps, even from trees that were brought down by Dutch elm disease.

Plant Constituents

The elm contains a substantial quantity of tannins, alkaloids, anthraquinones, and glucosides.

Traditional Uses

During the Middle Ages it was common for legal verdicts to be handed down outdoors beneath the foliage of an elm tree. Its size makes it a worthy competitor with the oak and chestnut.

Elm's diuretic and purifying properties were well known to our ancestors. They figured strongly in recipes of the Middle Ages for skin treatments, such as the following:

Place 10 grams of the bark in 2 liters of water. Allow it to boil for ten minutes, strain, then drink four cups daily.

The Gemmotherapy Remedy

The part of the plant used to make the gemmotherapy remedy is the bud.

Principal Action

Its draining action is one of its most commendable properties and makes this extract an excellent remedy for treating any problems affecting the skin. For this reason, elm is indicated in the treatment of eczema, acne, and herpes simplex outbreaks.

Secondary Action

Its purifying properties reduce the level of uric acid in the bloodstream, making it a potent weapon for treating gout. It also has an antidiarrheal action.

Fig Tree

Ficus carica

This tree is a native of Asia that can grow as tall as thirty feet, but is more often closer to fifteen feet. Its fruit, vaguely pear-shaped but considerably smaller than the pear, is harvested in late summer. This fruit has been used throughout recorded human history.

Plant Constituents

Figs contain 50 percent sugar, enzymes, flavonoids, and latex.

Traditional Uses

The fig played an important role in ancient traditions and mythology. It is cited quite frequently in the Bible, and allegedly Adam and Eve used a fig leaf to hide their nakedness.

In ancient Sparta, athletes consumed figs before physical contests and ordeals.

And according to some traditions, it was beneath a fig tree that Buddha received his illumination.

Plato called the fig the "philosopher's friend" because it appeared to sharpen the intellect and soothe the mind.

Fig seeds also contain a proven laxative action. The sap from the branches of the fig tree can eliminate warts and corns if applied on a regular basis, but can be an irritant to unblemished skin.

The Gemmotherapy Remedy

The part of the plant used to make the gemmotherapy remedy is the bud.

Principal Action

Gemmotherapy reveals the full range of the fig's healing potential. Fig tree buds demonstrate remarkable qualities for regulating the endocrine system and alleviating psychosomatic disorders. Figs are capable of acting on any symptoms of psycho-emotional origin, which makes them an excellent remedy for stress.

Because the stomach is the organ that bears the brunt of our emotions, which it symbolically digests (hence the popular expression "I cannot stomach that"), fig tree extract is the primary remedy prescribed in situations of emotional disturbance.

It is also an excellent remedy for herniated diaphragms, ulcers, gastritis, and colitis. It has a very visible positive effect on bulimia, which has its origins in emotion.

Secondary Action

Fig tree buds have a soothing and regulating action on the nervous system, one that is just as effective as that provided by pharmaceutical tranquilizers (without any of the side effects) and should be recommended for treating depression, spasmophilia, and sleep disorders. Fig tree bud extract is also quite effective against migraines.

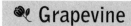 Grapevine

Vitis vinifera

The grapevine is a creeping, rambling bushy plant that exists in countless varieties. It prefers growing in limestone soil and gentle temperate climates.

Its hardy main stalk grows long branching stems that can sometimes attain lengths of thirty feet or more, which are more properly known as vine shoots. The leaves are heart-shaped and dentate; they have long green petioles and their undersides are downy. The flowers of this vine are small, green, and aromatic, and are arranged in clusters. The fruit of the vine is, of course, the grape.

Plant Constituents

Grapevines include a substantial amount of tannins, sugar, flavonoids (helpful for good blood circulation), and vitamins A, B, and C.

Traditional Uses

The origin of vine cultivation is lost in the depths of time. The legend that attributes the planting of the first grapevine to Noah suggests that this plant originated in Asia Minor. It was subsequently brought into Gaul by the Greeks sometime around 600 or 700 BCE. Naturalists throughout history have showered praise upon this plant and greatly praised its virtues and its fruit.

Bonum vinum leatifocat cor hominum, promises an ecclesiastical proverb, which translates to, "Good wine gladdens a person's heart."

In 1653 English physician Nicholas Culpeper recommended using the vine in mouthwashes, noting that the ashes of the vine shoots would make the teeth "white as snow." The antidiarrheal properties of the leaves of this plant have long been recognized.

Just as grape cures were recommended for purifying the body, Dr. Bach advised use of the vine in his flower therapy for rigid and proud individuals who abused their authority to grab more power. The

Grapevine remedy gives such individuals greater flexibility, allowing them to use their power not only in their own selfish interests, but for the good of all.

The Gemmotherapy Remedy

The part of the plant used to make the gemmotherapy remedy is the bud.

Principal Action

Grapevine is beneficial for the bloodstream, but the gemmotherapy form of grapevine reveals its most potent qualities in treating inflammations. This is why grapevine extract should be used when treating chronic rheumatic problems accompanied by deformities. Here again we find the doctrine of signatures at work, as the similarity between arthritic deformities and grapevine shoots is obvious.

Secondary Action

The grapevine extract also reveals an antifibrous action that is helpful for treating uterine fibroids and prostate adenoma. Grapevine appears to soften these growths.

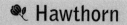 Hawthorn

Crataegus oxyacantha

The hawthorn shrub is often found in hedgerows, fields, and at the borders of woods in the temperate regions of the Northern Hemisphere.

Its flowering branches are cut in late spring and its bright red berries, sometimes known as "haws," are harvested at the beginning of autumn.

Plant Constituents

Flavonoids, coumarins, and vitamin C

Traditional Uses

The hawthorn has been regarded as a plant conferring protection—against a range of threats, from storms to vampires—for millennia.

The ancient Romans hung hawthorn branches on the cradles of newborns to protect them from illness. It also seems likely that the crown worn by Jesus Christ was woven from the branches of this bush.

Taking a more positive approach, in ancient Greek weddings the bride and groom each held several hawthorn flowers as a pledge for happiness and prosperity. This nuptial theme continued during the Middle Ages, when torches used to illuminate the nuptial chamber were made from hawthorn wood, and knights leaving for the Crusades would offer their ladies a hawthorn branch as a pledge of fidelity and a token of hope.

The hawthorn seems to have been a constant presence in human history, not only for its symbolic qualities but also for its therapeutic properties. Over the ages it has been used to combat anxiety, treat kidney problems, and most significantly, for its action on the cardiovascular system. Hawthorn tea (one teaspoon of flowers per cup, three times a day) is a proven regulator of blood pressure. A decoction of hawthorn has also been used to fight urine retention.

The Gemmotherapy Remedy

The part of the plant used to make the gemmotherapy remedy is the bud.

Principal Action

Gemmotherapy makes it possible to restore normal vascular and cardiac rhythm, whether caused by rhythm disorders (tachycardia, extrasystoles) or heart failure. This extract has a remarkable effect on arterial pressure, as hawthorn normalizes blood pressure, whether it is too high or too low. This action is much more rapid with the gemmotherapy extract than with traditional hawthorn preparations.

Secondary Action

Hawthorn is also used in the following capacities:

- It has a sedative effect on the nervous system and can be considered to be a tranquilizer, helpful in the treatment of depression as well as bulimia, which also makes it useful for treating weight issues.
- It addresses hyperthyroidism by slowing the activity of the thyroid.
- It has an important antisclerous property that makes hawthorn gemmotherapy extract a valid approach for the rejuvenation of all tissue.

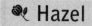 Hazel

Corylus avellana

The common hazel is a thick shrub native to Europe and western Asia. It typically grows twelve to fifteen feet tall, but can reach heights of fifty feet. It is commonly found in hedgerows, thickets, and wooded areas.

Its deciduous leaves are oval, heart-shaped at the base, and dentate. They grow in an alternating pattern and are slightly "hairy" when immature. Strangely enough, the female flowers, clustered in a kind of bud, appear in February before the leaves. Male flowers grow in September in the form of long yellow catkins hanging down from the branches.

Plant Constituents

The hazel tree contains essential oils, tannins, resins, wax, and vitamin C.

Traditional Uses

The Latin name, *Corylus,* comes from the Greek word *korus,* which means "helmet," because of the shape and hardness of hazelnut shells. The English name, hazel, derives from the German word for "bush," which is *hasel.*

Since ancient times, the hazelnut has been attributed with numerous qualities. Pliny, Virgil, and Cato, to mention only the most famous Latin authors with an opinion on this subject, praised its powers of rejuvenation and revitalization.

In the first century, Dioscorides recommended hazelnut as a remedy for coughs.

In the Middle Ages, Hildegard von Bingen, basing her prescription on the hazelnut's shape, or signature, recommended it as a treatment for impotence.

Hazelnuts were prescribed in the seventeenth century as a remedy against kidney and bile stones, and against nephritic pains.

The properties of the hazel tree have often been compared with those of "witch hazel," the Latin name of which is *Hamamelis*.

Hazel tree decoctions made from the bark of young branches or from the root were also used to fight fevers, as well as to sometimes treat grippe and pneumonia.

The oil from its kernel was successfully administered to get rid of tapeworms.

Finally, an infusion brewed from hazel leaves was used internally for cleansing and externally to assist scarring of wounds and ulcers.

The Gemmotherapy Remedy

The part of the plant used to make the gemmotherapy remedy is the bud.

Principal Action

When macerated in a gemmotherapy extract, the hazel tree bud does three important things:

- It acts on the pulmonary system in a way that is beneficial in treating emphysema and asthma.
- It accelerates the synthesis of white corpuscles in the bloodstream, which makes it valuable for treating leukemia and other illnesses that lower white corpuscle counts.
- It reverses the hardening of arterial blood vessels, therefore making this extract helpful in treating arteritis.

Secondary Action

The hazel tree bud extract soothes and restores the balance of the nervous system.

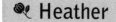 Heather

Calluna vulgaris

Heather is a small, low shrub with pink or violet flowers that grows in moors, marshlands, peat bogs, and some clearings.

Plant Constituents

Heather contains flavonoids, tannins, and ericodine (*erica* is Greek for "to break")

Traditional Uses

Heather flowers are essentially a urinary antiseptic that successfully treats bladder stones and cystitis, and the name of its primary alkaloid comes from its ability to break up bladder and kidney stones. It was recommended by the ancient Greek physician Galen for curing urinary and prostate problems. A decoction of the flowers is necessary for this treatment.

Dr. Bach recommended Heather for people who are continually seeking others' attention, talk constantly about themselves, and cannot tolerate being alone. People like this can be described as energy vampires who feed on the energy of those around them. Heather allows these people to refocus and regain self-esteem without constantly needing attention as a way to validate their lives.

The Gemmotherapy Remedy

The part of the plant used to make the gemmotherapy remedy is primarily the bud.

Principal Action

Heather's disinfecting effect on the urinary system is greatly amplified as compared to its traditional herbal use.

Secondary Action

Heather purifies and disinfects the bladder and bile ducts.

🌹 Hedge Maple

Acer campestre

This tree, a native of Asia, produces an extremely hard wood. It primarily grows in hedgerows and thickets on the borders of forests. Its height ranges from fifty to eighty feet.

Plant Constituents

This species of maple contains steroids, gums, glucides, and tannins.

Traditional Uses

Maple trees have played such an important role in Canada that a maple leaf appears on the Canadian flag, but other than as a syrup with digestive properties, it has scarcely been used for therapeutic purposes.

The Gemmotherapy Remedy

The part of the plant used to make the gemmotherapy remedy is the bud.

Principal Action

Maple buds have a tonic effect on digestion because they stimulate the gallbladder. They have a purifying effect on the kidneys due to the antispasmodic action they induce by relaxing the sphincter.

Secondary Action

Maple buds lower the rate of blood sugar, which makes this extract helpful in the treatment of certain kinds of diabetes.

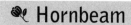 Hornbeam

Carpinus betulus

The hornbeam tree is primarily found in hedgerows and thickets. It is often grown as an ornamental tree in English gardens and for topiary in landscaping projects.

Plant Constituents

Hornbeam contains polysaccharides and an oil with properties that primarily affect the bloodstream.

Traditional Uses

The leaves and branches of hornbeam have been primarily employed for decorative ends; there has been very little used for medicinal purposes.

One exception is that Dr. Bach created a Bach Flower Remedy from hornbeam for those who suffer from "Monday morning blues" and are prematurely tired by the thought of the work in store for them during the coming week. Even the thought of starting a new week or going back to work after the weekend break prompts this individual to complain of feeling completely worn out and lacking energy.

In fact, what truly disturbs this individual is the idea of a new pace, and Hornbeam remedy supports the ability and strength to overcome what the person perceives to be an obstacle.

The Gemmotherapy Remedy

The part of the plant used to make the gemmotherapy remedy is the bud.

Principal Action

The gemmotherapy hornbeam extract has been shown to have an effect on blood, primarily targeting platelets.

Platelets in blood play a role in the phenomenon of coagulation, and in the immune and defense systems of the body. A normal adult count of platelets is 150,000 to 400,000 per microliter on average. If the number of platelets falls below this level, there is danger of hemorrhaging and the bursting of small blood vessels under the skin. The destruction of these small vessels is responsible for red or purple patches on the skin, a condition known as purpura (Latin for purple). Their appearance can be signs of a serious, even life-threatening disease.

Hornbeam is, therefore, an excellent remedy against hemorrhaging and can be used no matter what the cause, whether it is a wound, infection, pharmaceutical toxicity, or overuse of anticoagulant medication.

Secondary Action

Hornbeam also works on the hepatic level, respiratory system, and ORL (oto-rhino-laryngological system), which includes relieving sinus infections, rhinitis, and bronchitis.

❧ Horse Chestnut

Aesculus hippocastanum

A native of the forests of India and the Balkans, the horse chestnut is primarily grown today as an ornamental tree because of its flowers and fruit, which are not to be confused with the edible chestnuts they resemble.

Plant Constituents

The horse chestnut tree contains coumarins, such as esculoside; polysaccharides; tannins; and 2 percent essential oil.

Traditional Uses

Introduced into European medicine during the reign of King Louis XV of France (early seventeenth century), the horse chestnut is rightly considered to be a blood thinner and to have a tonic effect on the veins.

Because of the shape of its pointed spiny shells that contain a fruit similar to the chestnut, the theory of signatures has successfully recommended it as a remedy for hemorrhoids.

One old tradition recommends carrying one or two horse chestnuts next to your skin to prevent rheumatism, a condition that shows evidence of being caused by toxic elements in the blood.

The Gemmotherapy Remedy

The part of the plant used to make the gemmotherapy remedy is the bud.

Principal Action

Horse chestnut is used to stimulate vein and capillary circulation, which makes it helpful for the treatment of hemorrhoids and broken veins.

Secondary Action

This extract also demonstrates a decongestive effect around the lower pelvis (the prostate in men) and antiseptic properties that work on the bronchopulmonary apparatus. For this reason it is indicated in treatments against both prostatitis and bronchitis.

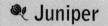 Juniper

Juniperus communis

Juniper is a thorny evergreen shrub that is sometimes classified as a member of the pine tree family. Its purple berries take two years to reach maturity. This tree is relatively small and more like a shrub, although it can reach heights of more than thirty feet. Its leaves are like needles.

Plant Constituents

The fruits are extremely rich in essential oil and contain more than sixty different constituent elements, including myrcene (from which they get their characteristic odor), terpenes, sugars, and resins.

Traditional Uses

Medicine has been relying on juniper since the dawn of time.

- Its berries have been used to perfume clear colorless brandy in Nordic countries, and in Finland it is a key ingredient in ale. However, the alcohol it is best known for flavoring is gin.
- A diuretic beverage obtained from its stems is useful in treating kidney stones.
- At one time its dried leaves were regularly cast into the hearth fire because of their reputation for cleansing the house, repelling plague, and driving away evil spirits. Juniper wood, meanwhile, was reputed to last for more than a century before it would start to rot. This is undoubtedly the reason Hannibal insisted that the beams for all the temples of Carthage be constructed from juniper wood.

The Gemmotherapy Remedy

The part of the plant used to make the gemmotherapy remedy is the young shoot.

Principal Action

This extract has a potent effect on the liver (particularly when combined with rosemary extract). It has proven itself to be effective in drainage of this organ, which it purifies and regenerates.

It can be used against all forms of hepatitis and all cases in which the liver and kidneys are overworked or overloaded, whether the cause is dietary or pharmaceutical.

Secondary Action

Juniper buds are a powerful diuretic with the power to dissolve most kidney stones.

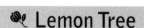 Lemon Tree

Citrus limonum

The lemon tree is a small, shrub-size tree that grows to about fifteen feet in height. Its origins are unknown, but it has been linked to both Iran and India. Lemon trees can grow only in subtropical regions and do best in coastal areas.

Its branches are long with fairly large, pale green, oval leaves, with a small winged petiole. Its flowers are extremely aromatic and have the distinction of being white on the inside and purple on the outside. This tree flowers for much of the year and is, in fact, the sole tree that is almost constantly bearing fruit, flowers, and leaves.

The fruit, as everyone knows, is an oblong, almost globular sphere that has a very attractive yellow color and extremely acidic juice.

Plant Constituents

Lemons are rich in mineral salts, gums, and glucides, and in vitamins A, C, PP (also known as niacin or B_3), and B.

Lemons also contain a very aromatic and bitter yellow-green essence that is highly antiseptic. This essence allows lemon juice to quickly kill cholera, diphtheria, and typhoid bacteria. In fifteen minutes, lemon juice will rid oysters and other crustaceans of 95 percent of their bacteria.

Traditional Uses

Because of their antiseptic and digestive properties, lemons have always been used extensively in kitchens as an addition to sauces, to enhance meats that are fatty or have been aged (or to mask the flavor of meat that has started to go bad), and in fish dishes.

There is also a remedy for obesity that consists of diluting the juice of three or four lemons with water, adding a little sugar, and drinking it on an empty stomach every morning for three weeks. In order to obtain the maximum amount of juice, the lemons should be placed in hot water for several minutes prior to squeezing.

Lemon has always been recognized as a formidable weapon against rheumatism and gout, as the citric acid it contains is a potent dissolver of uric acid. It also prevents scurvy and helps to prevent the common cold.

In the cosmetic realm, lemon juice applied to the face with a cotton swab every morning is generally very effective at improving the tone and color of the skin, as well as helping it relax. Similarly, lemon zest rubbed on the teeth will make them whiter and lemon juice will help to alleviate gingivitis. One caveat is that prolonged use will reduce the level of the teeth by eroding the enamel.

It can also be used to strengthen fingernails and soften the hands.

The Gemmotherapy Remedy

The part of the plant used to make the gemmotherapy remedy is the young shoot.

Principal Action

In its gemmotherapy form, the lemon tree reveals its remarkable properties as a blood thinning agent and those that are very active in the treatment of arteritis and varicose veins. This is evidence of its dual action on vein and artery circulation.

Secondary Action

It is also an excellent digestive tonic that should be prescribed for the treatment of all migraines of a digestive origin.

Lilac

Syringa vulgaris

Lilac is a shrub that generally grows an average of six feet high. It was originally native to Persia and cultivated as an ornamental plant because of its flowers and aroma. It flowers in April and May, and was introduced into western Europe in the late sixteenth century while practically retaining its Persian name: *lilak*.

Plant Constituents

Lilacs contain essential oils in their flowers, vitamin C in their leaves, and glucosides in their roots.

Traditional Uses

The lilac was brewed into a tea for treating rheumatism.

Its flowers, macerated in olive oil, were used in ancient times for massaging athletes. A recipe for this massage oil can still be found in some Russian villages. It is copied below:

> Macerate 100 grams of fresh flowers in one half liter of olive oil in a jar exposed to sunlight for fifteen days. Filter the oil and use it as a rub two times a day.

The Gemmotherapy Remedy

The part of the plant used to make the gemmotherapy remedy is the bud.

The gemmotherapy lilac extract shows evidence of significant action affecting the cardiovascular system, one which is not present in its traditional applications and extends far beyond its antirheumatic properties. In fact, lilac extract thins the blood and dilates the coronary arteries.

Principal Action

This extract has two properties that can be used for effective treatment of coronary disorders.

Secondary Action

It has significant antirheumatic properties.

❧ Lingonberry

Vaccinium vitis idaea

Lingonberry is a small evergreen shrub that grows around eight to eighteen inches tall, with green angular branches. It grows in the temperate and subarctic zones of the Northern Hemisphere, and its berries can be harvested from midsummer to early September.

Lingonberries were once used to dye cloth. Today they are more often used in jam and pastries, and as an accompaniment to game and red meat.

Plant Constituents

The berries contain 7 percent tannin, flavonoids, pectin, vitamin B_1, and carotene.

Traditional Uses

An extract made from the berry has been a long-standing remedy against dysentery. It can be drunk as a tea or applied to the stomach as a poultice.

Experiments performed at the beginning of the twenty-first century demonstrated that a culture of eberth bacteria (an agent responsible for spreading typhoid fever) would be sterilized in twenty-four hours by a decoction made from lingonberries.

The Gemmotherapy Remedy

The part of the plant used to make the gemmotherapy remedy is the young shoot, which should be harvested as soon as it appears for optimum results.

Principal Action

The gemmotherapy extract from lingonberries has properties that were never known or exploited in traditional healing preparations, and which are particularly potent for women. For example, lingonberry extract can be used for treating menstrual problems (irregularity, amenorrhea), menopause issues (hot flashes), fibroids, and ovarian cysts; and for postmenopausal women, this extract helps retain calcium in the bones, thus making it an important ally in the prevention and treatment of osteoporosis.

Secondary Action

Lingonberry is also used in the following capacities:

- *Digestive tract.* Lingonberry's beneficial properties for the intestinal organs are amplified in the gemmotherapy extract, making it a marvelous intestinal disinfectant in cases of constipation, spasmodic colitis, diarrhea, and problems with colon motility.
- *Kidney function.* The gemmotherapy extract has a disinfectant diuretic action that is helpful for eliminating oxalocalcic deposits (concretions) that are sometimes present in the kidneys.

  It also has a notable soothing effect on cystitis and a tonic effect on the prostate.
- *Osteoarticular system.* Lingonberry extract strengthens the bone and joint systems, and encourages greater mobility in the joints of both sexes.

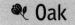 Oak

Quercus robur

This majestic tree was considered the most sacred of all trees by the Druids, and it still holds great symbolic value as the king of the forest and a symbol of power. It is one of the longest living of all trees, with some individual trees living for more than one thousand years. It is a large deciduous tree with lobed, almost sessile (attached directly at the base) leaves. Its fruit, the acorn, ripens in autumn.

Plant Constituents

The chief constituent elements of oak are tannins.

Traditional Uses

A decoction made from oak bark has long been used for soothing sore throats and treating tonsillitis and similar infections.

Its leaves, however, were steeped in honey-laced wine as a treatment for receding gums, a common complaint as early as Roman times, when oak leave decoctions were also used for vaginal baths to prevent or treat hemorrhaging.

Dr. Bach recommended Oak remedy to those who were overburdened with responsibility or carried too many heavy loads on their shoulders, psychologically speaking, taking on the problems of others to the point of exhaustion. This remedy supports them in remaining strong in their efforts, as well as in learning not to push themselves to the brink.

The Gemmotherapy Remedy

The part of the plant used to make the gemmotherapy remedy is the bud.

Principal Action

As shown by its shape, longevity, and symbolic potency, the oak is a remarkable tonic that can awaken an individual's natural healing abilities, making it recommended in the treatment of all lingering and chronic conditions that resist therapeutic treatment.

Secondary Action

Its tonic properties have a potent effect on the body's glandular system; this extract stimulates the ovaries for women and increases testosterone production in men.

It has a purifying action on the skin that can be helpful for treating recurring herpes outbreaks. It also tones the dental alveoli wall and the gums, just as it did in Roman times when it was used to combat receding gums and loose teeth.

Olive Tree

Olea europaea

Olives grow wild throughout the Mediterranean basin region, where they have been cultivated for centuries for their many nutritional and dietary qualities. They have been imported successfully into similar subtropical climates in North America (California), and into Australia, Chile, and New Zealand.

Plant Constituents

Olive oil contains 75 percent oleic acid, which is a monounsaturated fatty acid that has the ability to break down fat. It also contains vitamin E.

Traditional Uses

The olive tree has long been associated with numerous symbols for peace and victory, and even today, an olive branch appears on the United Nations flag. A crown woven from olive leaves was placed on the brows of the victors in the original Olympic Games of ancient Greece, where the tree was also considered to be a symbol for wisdom.

The olive has been friend, doctor, and sustenance for the people of the Mediterranean basin since time immemorial. Its particularly hardy wood can be used as a building material and for heating. Its leaves have healing properties and its fruit (the olive), whether intact or pressed into an oil, has fed and kept people healthy.

Olive tree leaves were used to disinfect wounds and have a similarly remarkable detoxifying effect on the digestive system, which they encourage to drain. A decoction of olive leaves is also recommended for treating diabetes.

For liver problems or colitis, it has long been recommended to swallow a tablespoon of cold-pressed olive oil on an empty stomach; and relief for liver or kidney crises can be quickly obtained by drinking a small glass of olive oil every half hour.

In external application, two tablespoons of olive oil blended into a beaten egg white will provide skin relief for burns and sunburn (however, extreme burns may heat the oil and aggravate the problem).

Dr. Bach recommended Olive remedy to counter the physical and mental exhaustion that follows a long illness or protracted effort.

The Gemmotherapy Remedy

The part of the plant used to make the gemmotherapy remedy is the young shoot.

Principal Action

In the extract form, olive's digestive action is not the most important health benefit it provides. Rather, it is its potent effect on cerebral circulation that makes olive extract very useful for problems caused by aging and for the aftereffects of some forms of cerebral palsy. Use of this extract has made gradual restoration of adequate brain function possible.

Secondary Action

The olive's ability to deal with excess lipids in the blood is apparent. The gemmotherapy olive extract dissolves cholesterol and provides the appropriate balance of phospholipids necessary for proper brain functioning. Similarly, this extract also possesses a slight hypotensive effect that is useful for treating high blood pressure.

Raspberry Bush

Rubus idaeus

The raspberry bush is a perennial low-lying plant bearing biennial stems from its root system. It is vegetative in its first season and produces fruit only in its second year; however, this maceration uses first year shoots. Raspberry bushes are chiefly found along garden hedges and in forest clearings.

Plant Constituents

Raspberries mainly contain sugars and vitamins A, B_1, and C.

Traditional Uses

A decoction from the leaves has long been used to make poultices for treating skin rashes and eye inflammation. A tea brewed from the leaves was recommended for treating flu in earlier times, and was also used as a mouthwash for throat ailments during the Middle Ages. The leaves were also used in various folk medicine traditions to treat gingivitis, anemia, and diarrhea.

The ingested berries have always been considered fortifying. A vinegar made from raspberries was also reputed to prevent plague.

The Gemmotherapy Remedy

The part of the plant used to make the gemmotherapy remedy is the young shoot.

Principal Action

Gemmotherapy significantly amplifies the existing healing properties of raspberry and has also revealed new ones. Because of its resemblance to an ovary bearing numerous oocytes, raspberry extract is the preeminent remedy for treating the female hormonal system. It stimulates the release of estrogens and progesterone, and regulates menstrual flow, thus alleviating menstrual cramps.

It is also a valuable uterine antispasmodic for treating bleeding.

Secondary Action

Raspberry extract also seems to have an effect on the respiratory system, and helps in countering allergies.

🌹 Rosemary

Rosmarinus officinalis

Rosemary is a native of the Mediterranean basin, where it grows abundantly in the wild. It is a small, aromatic woody herb with narrow green leaves and pale blue or mauve flowers.

Plant Constituents

Rosemary contains an essential oil rich in borneol and camphor, flavonoids, tannins, and terpenes.

Traditional Uses

Rosemary has long been used to stimulate memory and attention. It was once burned in workplaces to increase cerebral circulation through its stimulating properties.

The Romans turned to it for treating hair loss, as rosemary appeared to stimulate new hair growth by its stimulation of the irrigation of the scalp.

Rosemary was one of the ingredients in the famous "Queen of Hungary water," which had a reputation for conferring undying beauty on those who used it.

Rosemary has long been used in cooking, not only for flavor but for the way it stimulates digestion.

The Gemmotherapy Remedy

The part of the plant used to make the gemmotherapy remedy is the young shoot.

Principal Action

The extract's hepatic detoxification action and its ability to stimulate bile release is much greater than that of the entire plant. Gemmotherapy rosemary extract is the preferred remedy for treating liver problems. It can also be used with juniper extract for an even more potent effect.

Secondary Action

Rosemary extract is mentally stimulating, which may be a consequence of its hepatic action. Because the liver has always been closely tied to a person's emotional and mental state, a French folk saying equates worrying with making bile, so that when rosemary stimulates and restores normal hepatic function, it also improves mental function.

In the case of rosemary extract, doses should begin small and be increased gradually to the recommended levels, in order to avoid an overly intense action on the liver. Too much, too soon could lead to the body being temporarily inundated by its own toxins.

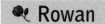 Rowan

Sorbus domestica

The rowan, or service tree, is a small tree with white flowers and reddish-orange fruit that prefers to grow in wooded areas. Birds are extremely fond of it, which has earned it the nickname of "bird tree" in some regions.

Plant Constituents

The pear-shaped fruit of the rowan tree contains tannins that contribute to its astringent properties, as well as sorbitol and high levels of vitamin C.

The seeds contain glucosides that produce the toxin prussic acid when they decompose.

Traditional Uses

Because of its astringent qualities, the fruit of the rowan tree was formerly used in the forms of infusions and jellies to treat vomiting and diarrhea. The fruit also revealed itself to be useful in treating hemorrhoids, often a consequence of diarrhea.

The Gemmotherapy Remedy

The part of the plant used to make the gemmotherapy remedy is the bud.

Principal Action

The extract increases the potency of the traditionally used rowan tree tea, and is particularly effective for veins and capillaries.

Secondary Action

Rowan tree bud extract works very effectively on the extremities of some individuals (cold feet and hands), and can also be extremely helpful for treating ringing in the ears (tinnitus).

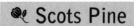

Scots Pine

Pinus sylvestris

Scots pine is an evergreen coniferous tree with bark that is dark gray near the base of the tree and reddish-orange-brown toward the top. This needle-bearing tree can reach heights of 150 feet. There are more than eighty species in the botanical literature, but recent research has consolidated the number down to four. Its therapeutic benefits were discovered very early by our ancestors.

Plant Constituents

Pine contains an essential oil composed of alphapineme and resins that are responsible for both its aroma and its healing properties.

Traditional Uses

The characteristic odor and its effect on breathing are the most visible evidence of the pine tree's beneficial properties for the respiratory system. For this reason, the same resin that is used to make turpentine and pine oil is also a key ingredient in many disinfectants.

Dr. Bach recommended Pine remedy for treating excessive feelings of guilt. It was his prescription of choice for individuals who were highly self-critical and always blamed themselves for the sins of others. Pine remedy enables these individuals to raise their level of awareness and overcome this often inappropriate sense of guilt.

The Gemmotherapy Remedy

The part of the plant used to make the gemmotherapy remedy is the bud.

Principal Action

Scots pine gemmotherapy extract shows evidence of potent action on the osteoarticular system, as well as a strong ability to restore mineral content to the body. This makes this extract an essential remedy in the treatment of joints afflicted with osteoarthritis. It is also very helpful for treating osteoporosis.

Secondary Action

Pine extract exhibits a tonic effect on the mind, as well as a stimulant effect on the respiratory tract.

🌷 Sequoia
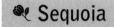

Sequoia gigantea

A native of California, the sequoia has been gradually introduced into other regions of the world for its ornamental qualities. It is a majestic tree that can grow taller than 350 feet and live for thousands of years. California has entire forests of these beautiful trees that have become a huge tourist attraction, especially in the fall.

Plant Constituents

This tree contains tannins, resins, and flavonoids.

Traditional Uses

Sequoia, for obvious reasons, had little therapeutic use in European traditional and folk medicine, but Native Americans in what is now northern California were very familiar with its tonic effects.

In spring they collected the sap by making slashes in the trunk. They then mixed this resin with honey and ingested it for its reinvigorating qualities.

The Gemmotherapy Remedy

The part of the plant used to make the gemmotherapy remedy is the young shoot.

Principal Action

Its primary properties reflect Native American traditional use of this tree insofar as it is a stimulant for the hormonal system. This property makes sequoia the best remedy for providing energy, as well as a preeminent antiaging supplement.

Sequoia increases sperm production in men because of its decongestant effect on the prostate. For women of childbearing age it restores normal menstrual cycles, and for older women it facilitates the transitional stage of menopause.

Secondary Action

Sequoia extract restores and retains mineral content in the body and encourages hepatic draining, as part of its overall tonic effect.

&ℓ Silver Linden

Tilia tomentosa

Silver linden (known as silver lime in the United Kingdom) is a native of Europe, where it grows wild and is also cultivated. It is a deciduous tree that can grow anywhere, and its mature height ranges from 70- to 110-feet tall. During the summer its blossoms are harvested for making tea.

Plant Constituents

Silver linden's leaves and blossoms contain 3 percent mucilage, 1 percent essential oil, and flavonoids that have a beneficial effect on blood circulation.

Traditional Uses

Silver linden was regarded as so valuable in the seventeenth century that a decree was enacted ordering the planting of these trees alongside all roads, with their harvest reserved for hospital use in treating the sick.

Silver linden has always been regarded in all its forms (tea, bath, decoction) as a sedative that relaxes the nervous system and encourages sleep.

The Gemmotherapy Remedy

The part of the plant used to make the gemmotherapy remedy is the bud.

Principal Action

The bud extract has a soothing effect on the nervous system, which is why it is recommended for combating all kinds of sleep disorders and insomnia, as well as being a potent remedy for anxiety.

Like the fig tree extract, silver linden is one of the most effective plant-based tranquilizers available.

Secondary Action

It increases the kidney's diuresis function, which makes it a valuable adjunct to treatments for kidney, liver, and rheumatic problems.

❧ Tamarind

Tamarix gallica

The tamarind tree is native to Africa, but it was introduced into India so long ago that it is commonly reported as originating there. The tree grows as tall as sixty-five feet and has pinnate leaves with opposite leaflets. The yellow flowers grow in clumps and its fruits are encased in pods.

Plant Constituents

Tamarind fruits contain 16 to 17 percent citric acid (vitamin C), salicylic acid, nicotine acid, potassium, and mineral salts.

Traditional Uses

Sailors once ate tamarind fruits regularly while at sea as a means of preventing scurvy, and returning navigators introduced the fruit into fifteenth-century Europe.

Tamarind has a reputation for helping digestion and having a mild laxative effect. It is still a major culinary ingredient in Indian chutneys, as well as in such English products as Worcestershire sauce.

The leaves were traditionally used in parts of Southeast Asia to brew a tea as a remedy for malaria. It was also used to relieve sore throats and as a compress to cool high body temperature. It is a primary component of the ayurvedic pharmacopoeia.

The Gemmotherapy Remedy

The part of the plant used to make the gemmotherapy remedy is the young shoot.

Principal Action

The extract displays properties that were little known and little used in traditional folk medicine. These properties increase bone marrow and stimulate the production of platelets and red blood cells.

This makes it extremely useful for the treatment of anemia, as it increases the size and number of these red blood cells. It is also effective for treating problems with blood coagulation.

Secondary Action

Tamarind extract stimulates appetite and improves digestion and intestinal transit. It is likely that these actions are partially responsible for its popularity as a cooking ingredient.

🌹 Wayfaring Tree

Viburnum lantana

Wayfaring tree is a sturdy shrub producing creamy white flowers and bright orange-red berries that turn a deep blue-black color as they mature. This potentially invasive plant grows up to sixteen feet in the wooded areas of the central and northeastern portions of the United States, as well as in Europe, North Africa, and Asia.

Plant Constituents

This shrub contains coumarins, the glucoside salicine, an essential oil, and tannins. Because it contains salicine, the use of wayfaring tree is, like white willow, contraindicated for those who are allergic to acetylsalicylic acid.

Traditional Uses

The wayfaring tree was mainly used by Native Americans, who ate its fruits as a remedy for dysentery.

Starting in the nineteenth century in Europe, the bark of this plant was employed with some success for its antispasmodic properties on the colon and uterus.

The Gemmotherapy Remedy

The part of the plant used to make the gemmotherapy remedy is the bud.

Principal Action

The extract reveals a pulmonary action that was not evident in other preparations. This effect is demonstrated by its ability to relax the autonomic respiratory system, which makes it extremely useful for treating spasmodic rhinitis and non-infectious bronchitis.

Secondary Action

Wayfaring tree extract also displays a relaxing effect on the autonomic elements of the ORL (oto-rhino-laryngology) system. This preparation can also slow activity of the thyroid, making it very valuable in the treatment of hyperthyroidism.

Of equal significance is its effect on the skin's ability to eliminate toxins, which makes it useful for treating chronic dermatosis.

❧ White Willow

Salix alba

Willow trees grow throughout the wetter regions of North America, western Asia, and Europe. This large deciduous tree is highly ornamental with the bizarre distinction of extremely small flowers encased in catkins.

Plant Constituents

The essential components of white willow are salicylic acid and tannins.

Traditional Uses

Willow is the ancestor of aspirin and has been known since ancient times for three healing benefits:

- Reduces fever
- Analgesic action
- Soothes and relaxes

This was why Dioscorides in the first century CE recommended eating willow leaves crushed with a little pepper and steeped in wine to soothe lumbar pain.

Endowed with astringent properties, white willow was also used to treat internal hemorrhages. And because it reduces perspiration, it was once used to alleviate hot flashes caused by menopause.

But it was not until the end of the nineteenth century that Bayer made his discovery concerning salicylic acid and white willow bark, which led to these properties being exploited in the now common form of aspirin.

Dr. Bach recommended White Willow remedy for those individuals who were prone to feeling bitterness and resentment, and who felt they were victimized by others. This remedy enables them to take responsibility for their feelings and to then analyze their experiences more objectively.

The Gemmotherapy Remedy

The part of the plant used to make the gemmotherapy remedy is the bud.

Principal Action

The anti-inflammatory and analgesic properties displayed by the typical herbal remedies using this plant are amplified in the extract. Most importantly, unlike aspirin, the extract of white willow bud does not thin the blood (and so prevents hemorrhaging), and does not irritate the mucous membrane lining of the stomach. It should be noted that white willow extract is contraindicated for anyone allergic to aspirin.

Secondary Action

The extract also includes soothing properties and is known for its use in anti-acne preparations.

❧ Wild or Dog Rose

Rosa canina

Wild Rose is a climbing plant that bears red or white flowers followed by red fruits (rose hips). It generally grows on the borders of hedgerows and thickets. It earned its Latin name, *Rosa canina,* from the fact that its root had the reputation for healing rabies and was used to treat dog bites in ancient times.

Plant Constituents

Rose hips are extremely rich in vitamin C (4.25 percent of total weight), and in vitamins A, B1, B2, P, and K. They are also rich in citric acid and carotenoids, and high in some antioxidants.

Traditional Uses

During the Middle Ages the fruit of the wild rose was a highly sought delicacy for its slightly acidic flavor and its nutritive qualities.

The hairy pith from the fruit, when applied to the skin, can cause a very unpleasant rash—hence many folk names referred to its itching qualities. However, it was also reputed to be an ideal antidote for parasitical intestinal worms. For example, fifteen grams of this down mixed with honey and ingested on an empty stomach proved to kill these worms immediately, without causing any intestinal distress.

The dried and powdered seeds of this plant reputedly were able to dissolve kidney stones.

The Gemmotherapy Remedy

The part of the plant used to make the gemmotherapy remedy is the young shoot.

Principal Action

The gemmotherapy preparation of wild rose has a potent effect on the immune system, especially in the ear, nose, and throat. This is why it is the extract of choice for certain conditions to which children are particularly susceptible, especially in winter, such as sore throats, colds, earaches, and tonsillitis.

Secondary Action

Because of its ability to strengthen the body's defenses, wild rose is very effective in treating infections, particularly those affecting the colon, and for its antirheumatic action.

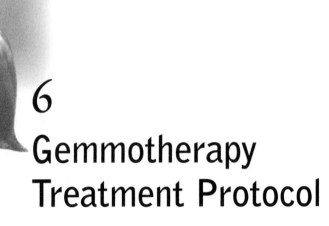

6
Gemmotherapy Treatment Protocol

Every illness is the consequence of an internal disorder, the origin of which can be traced back to a toxic state caused by external factors (dietary, respiratory, or pharmaceutical) or endogenous factors, such as emotions. This is why all treatment methods must first cleanse the body by triggering the drainage of toxins, before mounting an effort to restore it to optimum health.

In the same way that drainpipes evacuate excess water from a sink, the lymph system, which is the body's drainage system, collects excess fluid from throughout the body and conveys it through a series of small vessels and the lymph nodes (where it is purified) back into the bloodstream. Because this system transports both toxins and nutrients, it occasionally becomes congested. Gemmotherapy's high-powered concentrates provide an efficient way of reopening these passages.

In all cases and phases of treatment, the dosages recommended in this chapter will vary depending on the individual case and gemmotherapy extract selected. Only one type of formulation should be used for each dose: D1 homeopathic dilution, or full-strength concentrated extract, or oral spray.

DRAINAGE OF TOXINS

As we saw earlier, there are many clinical applications of gemmotherapy available, but in order to clear the body before beginning treatment, every protocol using gemmotherapy should start with two gemmotherapy draining formulas to perform a general purification of the body. Only then should treatment proceed with extracts that target the specific illness.

- The first gemmotherapy drainage formula has a base of birch extract, since birch is the preeminent purifier of the body.
- The second gemmotherapy drainage formula is fig (the best psychosomatic remedy), or black currant in the event of an allergy.

In order to fully detoxify and cleanse the body, the patient should take the prescribed extracts in the amounts and times outlined below.

Morning Protocol: Birch

After rising in the morning, take the recommended dose of one of the following forms of birch extract.

D1 homeopathic strength: 50 to 100 drops in water
Full-strength concentrated extract: 10 drops in water
Oral spray: 3 sprayings

Bedtime Protocol: Fig

At bedtime, take the recommended dose of one of the following forms of fig extract. This remedy is especially effective for detoxification related to psychosomatic problems.

D1 homeopathic strength: 50 to 100 drops in water
Full-strength concentrated extract: 10 drops in water
Oral spray: 3 sprayings

Alternate: Black Currant

If the patient has allergies, black currant can be used at bedtime in place of fig using one of the following forms:

D1 homeopathic strength: 50 to 100 drops in water

Full-strength concentrated extract: 10 drops in water

Oral spray: 3 sprayings

This draining period should continue for a month. Once the body has been thoroughly detoxified, attention can be turned to the specific organ systems that are diseased or dysfunctional.

APPLYING GEMMOTHERAPY REMEDIES USING REFLEXOLOGY

Gemmotherapy extracts may also be applied cutaneously. In addition to being one of the body's major elimination organs, the skin is also one of its major means of absorbing substances into the body. Modern science has taken advantage of this with the use of skin patches.

The body also has sensitive areas known as reflex zones; when stimulated, one of these zones can trigger a healing or regulating action in another part of the body, sometimes quite removed. These zones have been meticulously mapped out in the therapy known as reflexology or reflextherapy, and are mostly found on the feet and around the ears.

The application of a gemmotherapy extract on the zone corresponding to the organ or body function requiring treatment will have a noticeably amplified effect compared to that usually resulting from pressure massage.

To prepare the application, the following is required:

100 drops of D1 maceration or 20 drops of the concentrated maceration blended into 250 grams (a little less than nine ounces) of a neutral base substance such as a natural skin cream, or beeswax and olive oil

This ointment can then be applied to the zones traditionally massaged to treat their corresponding areas. The most important reflexology zones are located on the feet and ears, which is where the gemmotherapy ointment should be applied.

REFLEXOLOGY CORRESPONDENCES

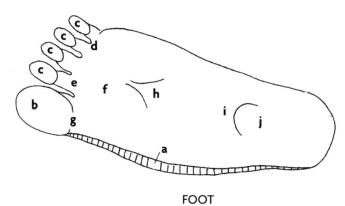

FOOT

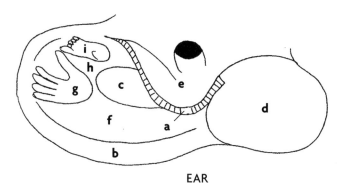

EAR

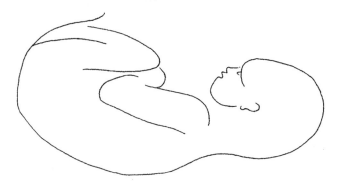

On the Foot:
a. spinal column
b. top of the head
c. brain, sinus
d. ears
e. eyes
f. chest, lungs, heart, solar plexus
g. throat
h. waist (liver, stomach, spleen, pancreas)
i. middle abdomen (adrenal glands, kidneys, small intestine, large intestine)
j. lower abdomen (colon, bladder, sex organs, rectum)

On the Ear:
a. spinal column
b. spinal cord
c. ribs
d. brain and skull
e. organs (lungs, heart, stomach, intestines, kidneys)
f. arms
g. hands
h. pelvis, legs
i. feet

Circulatory and Cardiovascular System

The circulatory system consists of the heart, blood, and blood vessels. The heart pumps the blood, which transports oxygen and essential nutrients out through the arteries to the organs. Systemic and pulmonary veins return the blood to the heart; systemic veins go directly to the heart from the body, and pulmonary veins convey oxygenated blood from the lungs to the heart.

The most important gemmotherapy extract for treating disorders of this system is hawthorn. Its use is indicated for:

- *Heart problems, tired cardiac muscle, heart failure.* Hawthorn is an excellent heartbeat regulator. It gives tone to the myocardium, especially in the left side of the heart, and has a soothing action on all cardiac-related chest pains. (It may also be necessary to prescribe a diuretic, such as ash, to accompany the hawthorn extract and lessen the burden placed on the heart function.)

- *Palpitations, tachycardia, and rhythmic disorders.* For these kinds of disorders, hawthorn can be combined with the anxiolytic (anti-anxiety) action of silver linden.

- *Coronary failure.* Lilac can be combined with hawthorn to treat coronary spasms and the arteriosclerosis that is often present.

- *Blood pressure problems.* Hawthorn has a dual action on blood pressure problems; it can lower the rate for someone experiencing high blood pressure, or raise the pressure of an individual suffering from low blood pressure. It is considered to be normotensive, meaning it establishes normal blood pressure.

- *Varicose veins, phlebitis, and hemorrhoids.* Rowan can be combined with hawthorn to treat problems related to vein circulation, particularly the cellular walls of the veins. Horse chestnut is indicated for problems in the lower pelvis. Chestnut acts on the lymphatic vessels, and lymphatic circulation plays a collateral role in varicose veins. Lemon tree is advised for its blood thinning effect. Varicose ulcers, which are painful and extremely difficult to remedy, can be effectively treated with the three gemmotherapy extracts of rowan, chestnut, and walnut.

- *Blood disorders.* For blood coagulation, repeated episodes of bleeding due to a low blood platelet count, or a reduction in white or red blood cells (lymphocytosis or leucocytosis), the following bud extracts offer equally valuable treatments: bloodtwig dogwood for cases of lowered platelet count, tamarind for cases involving red blood cells, and grapevine for cases involving white blood cells.

Tired Cardiac Muscle

Morning Protocol: Hawthorn

After rising in the morning, take the recommended dose of one of the following forms of hawthorn extract.

> *D1 homeopathic strength:* 50 drops in water
> *Full-strength concentrated extract:* 5 drops in water (increase this by one drop a day to 15 drops)
> *Oral spray:* 3 sprayings

Evening Protocol: Ash

At bedtime, take the recommended dose of one of the following forms of ash extract.

> *D1 homeopathic strength:* 50 drops in water
> *Full-strength concentrated extract:* 10 drops in water
> *Oral spray:* 3 sprayings

Heart Failure—Pre–Heart Attack State

Morning and Evening Protocol: Lilac

After rising in the morning and before bedtime, take the recommended dose of one of the following forms of lilac extract.

> *D1 homeopathic strength:* 50 drops in water
> *Full-strength concentrated extract:* 10 drops in water
> *Oral spray:* 3 sprayings

High Blood Pressure

Morning Protocol: Hawthorn

After rising in the morning, take the recommended dose of one of the following forms of hawthorn extract.

D1 homeopathic strength: 150 drops in water
Full-strength concentrated extract: 5 to 15 drops in water
Oral spray: 3 sprayings

Evening Protocol: Silver Linden

At bedtime, take the recommended dose of one of the following forms of silver linden extract.

D1 homeopathic strength: 150 drops in water
Full-strength concentrated extract: 15 drops in water
Oral spray: 3 sprayings

Vein Circulatory Disorders

Morning Protocol: Horse Chestnut and Rowan

After rising in the morning, take the recommended combined dose of one of the following forms of horse chestnut and rowan extracts.

D1 homeopathic strength: 50 drops each in a glass of water
Full-strength concentrated extract: 15 drops each in a glass of water
Oral spray: 3 sprayings of each

Evening Protocol: Chestnut

At bedtime, take the recommended dose of one of the following forms of chestnut extract.

D1 homeopathic strength: 50 drops in water
Full-strength concentrated extract: 10 drops in water
Oral spray: 3 sprayings

Blood Disorders: Platelet Issues

Morning and Evening Protocol: Bloodtwig Dogwood

After rising in the morning and again before bedtime, take the recommended dose of one of the following forms of bloodtwig dogwood extract.

D1 homeopathic strength: 150 drops in water

Full-strength concentrated extract: 15 drops in water

Oral spray: 3 sprayings

Blood Disorders: Cases Involving Red Blood Cells

Morning and Evening Protocol: Tamarind

After rising in the morning and again before bedtime, take the recommended dose of one of the following forms of tamarind extract.

D1 homeopathic strength: 150 drops in water

Full-strength concentrated extract: 15 drops in water

Oral spray: 3 sprayings

Blood Disorders: Cases Involving White Blood Cells

Morning and Evening Protocol: Grapevine

After rising in the morning and again before bedtime, take the recommended dose of one of the following forms of grapevine extract.

D1 homeopathic strength: 150 drops in water

Full-strength concentrated extract: 15 drops in water

Oral spray: 3 sprayings

&\ The Respiratory System and the Oto-rhino-laryngology (ORL) System

Our lungs absorb air with every inhalation, thereby incorporating the gaseous elements we need to sustain life; and with every exhalation, they expel those substances that no longer serve any purpose for the body.

Breathing is an autonomic process that starts in the nose and conveys oxygen to the lungs by way of the larynx and bronchial tubes. It is not news to anyone that this phenomenon is absolutely essential to life, as no one can survive for more than three minutes without breathing.

There are three categories of disorders that affect the ear, nose, and throat system and the pulmonary region: infectious diseases, allergies, and troubles caused by the ossification of the respiratory system (this generally means respiratory failure, as exemplified in such diseases as emphysema and chronic bronchitis).

- *Infectious diseases.* Gemmotherapy is extremely valuable for treating diseases of this nature because it addresses lingering infections commonly treated with antibiotic medications that have a number of undesirable side effects when used over a period of time. The side effects are themselves often extremely resistant to treatment.

  Common childhood illnesses (most often occurring in winter), such as colds, flu, earaches, sinusitis, and bronchitis, can be successfully treated with wild rose, birch, hornbeam, and black currant macerations. In addition, gemmotherapy extracts made from macerated grapevine and walnut are extremely useful for treating sore throats in both children and adults.

- *Allergies.* Whether it is a chronic case of allergic rhinitis or asthma, there are two gemmotherapy extracts that have proved their great worth for dealing with these common disorders: Black currant has anti-inflammatory action and stimulates the adrenal glands, which encourages the production of antiallergenic cortisol; and wayfaring tree has a sedative effect on the autonomic pulmonary system and helps restore respiratory function.

- *Ossification of the respiratory system (emphysema and chronic bronchitis).* Hazel extract restores the elasticity of pulmonary tissue and can be given in combination with black currant for its anti-inflammatory properties, and with horse chestnut.

Throat Infections in Children

Morning Protocol: Wild Rose

After rising in the morning, take the recommended dose of one of the following forms of wild rose extract.

D1 homeopathic strength: 50 drops in a glass of water
Full-strength concentrated extract: 10 drops in a glass of water
Oral spray: 3 sprayings

Evening Protocol: Black Currant

At bedtime, take the recommended dose of one of the following forms of black currant extract.

D1 homeopathic strength: 50 drops in a glass of water
Full-strength concentrated extract: 15 drops in a glass of water
Oral spray: 3 sprayings

Sinusitis and Ear Inflammation

Morning Protocol: Black Currant

After rising in the morning, take the recommended dose of one of the following forms of black currant extract.

D1 homeopathic strength: 150 drops in a glass of water
Full-strength concentrated extract: 15 drops in a glass of water
Oral spray: 3 sprayings

Evening Protocol: Hornbeam

At bedtime, take the recommended dose of one of the following forms of hornbeam extract.

D1 homeopathic strength: 150 drops in a glass of water

Full-strength concentrated extract: 15 drops in a glass of water
Oral spray: 3 sprayings

Chronic Bronchitis

This condition calls for three gemmotherapy remedies, one each at morning, noon, and bedtime.

Morning Protocol: Black Currant
After rising in the morning, take the recommended dose of one of the following forms of black currant extract.

D1 homeopathic strength: 150 drops in a glass of water
Full-strength concentrated extract: 15 drops in a glass of water
Oral spray: 3 sprayings

Noon Protocol: Hornbeam
Before your noon meal, take the recommended dose of one of the following forms of black currant extract.

D1 homeopathic strength: 50 drops in a glass of water
Full-strength concentrated extract: 10 drops in a glass of water
Oral spray: 3 sprayings

Evening Protocol: Walnut
At bedtime, take the recommended dose of one of the following forms of walnut extract.

D1 homeopathic strength: 150 drops in a glass of water
Full-strength concentrated extract: 15 drops in a glass of water
Oral spray: 3 sprayings

Asthma

Morning Protocol: Black Currant
After rising in the morning, take the recommended dose of one of the following forms of black currant extract.

D1 homeopathic strength: 100 drops in a glass of water
Full-strength concentrated extract: 15 drops in a glass of water
Oral spray: 3 sprayings

Evening Protocol: Wayfaring Tree

At bedtime, take the recommended dose of one of the following forms of wayfaring tree extract.

D1 homeopathic strength: 100 drops in a glass of water
Full-strength concentrated extract: 15 drops in a glass of water
Oral spray: 3 sprayings

Emphysema

Morning Protocol: Hazel

After rising in the morning, take the recommended dose of one of the following forms of hazel extract.

D1 homeopathic strength: 150 drops in a glass of water
Full-strength concentrated extract: 15 drops in a glass of water
Oral spray: 3 sprayings

Evening Protocol: Black Currant

At bedtime, take the recommended dose of one of the following forms of black currant extract.

D1 homeopathic strength: 150 drops in a glass of water
Full-strength concentrated extract: 15 drops in a glass of water
Oral spray: 3 sprayings

❧ The Digestive System

The digestive process starts in the mouth with the act of chewing food. It continues in the esophagus as food passes through on its way to the stomach, where digestive juices from the liver and pancreas break down the ingested food.

This broken down food matter then becomes the responsibility of the small intestine, which completes digestion. The process is finally concluded in the colon with the rejection of wastes that have been created.

Gemmotherapy can address all the disorders of the digestive system.

- *Mouth.* Bleeding gums, loosening teeth, dental abscesses, and pulpitis (inflammation of dental pulp resulting from tooth decay and other trauma) can all be treated by a combination of birch and oak extracts. These two extracts will aid the gums' ability to scar and give tone to alveoli ligaments.
- *Stomach.* Whether the disorder is gastritis, a hiatal hernia, digestive distress involving regurgitation, or ulcers, there are three extracts that have proven to be essential for providing treatment: fig, black currant, and silver linden.

  When one has grasped just how important a role the mind plays in the well-being of the stomach, it is easy to understand why extracts made from these three buds are so important.
- *Liver.* Rosemary and juniper have proven their mettle as the best remedies here by reason of their protective properties and their ability to repair hepatic cells.
- *Intestinal region.* Lingonberry extract is indicated in all cases, whether the difficulty is diarrhea, constipation, or spasms. This is because of its dual action that stimulates evacuation in the case of constipation and restrains it when the problem is diarrhea. This biphasic action also has a beneficial effect on spasmodic colitis.

Receding Gums (Periodontitis)

Morning Protocol: Birch

After rising in the morning, take the recommended dose of one of the following forms of birch extract.

D1 homeopathic strength: 150 drops in a glass of water

Full-strength concentrated extract: 15 drops in a glass of water

Oral spray: 3 sprayings

Evening Protocol: Oak

At bedtime, take the recommended dose of one of the following forms of oak extract.

D1 homeopathic strength: 150 drops in a glass of water

Full-strength concentrated extract: 15 drops in a glass of water

Oral spray: 3 sprayings

Gastritis, Hernias, Ulcers, and Acid Reflux

Morning Protocol: Fig and Black Currant

After rising in the morning, take the recommended dose of one of the following forms of fig and black currant extracts.

D1 homeopathic strength: 150 drops each combined in a glass of water

Full-strength concentrated extract: 15 drops each in a glass of water

Oral spray: 3 sprayings of each

Evening Protocol: Silver Linden

At bedtime, take the recommended dose of one of the following forms of silver linden extract.

D1 homeopathic strength: 150 drops in a glass of water

Full-strength concentrated extract: 15 drops in a glass of water

Oral spray: 3 sprayings

Liver Dysfunction

Depending on the case, problems of this nature are usually treated with two gemmotherapy extracts in the morning, rosemary and olive; and juniper in the evening.

Morning Protocol: Rosemary and Olive

After rising in the morning, take the recommended dose of one of the following forms of rosemary and olive extracts.

D1 homeopathic strength: 150 drops of rosemary extract and 100 drops of olive in a glass of water

Full-strength concentrated extract: 15 drops rosemary and ten drops olive in a glass of water

Oral spray: 3 sprayings of each

Evening Protocol: Juniper

At bedtime, take the recommended dose of one of the following forms of juniper extract.

D1 homeopathic strength: 100 drops in a glass of water

Full-strength concentrated extract: 5 drops in a glass of water

Oral spray: 3 sprayings

Intestinal Problems

For diarrhea and constipation specifically, lingonberry and walnut are especially effective.

Morning Protocol: Lingonberry

After rising in the morning, take the recommended dose of one of the following forms of lingonberry extract.

D1 homeopathic strength: 100 drops in a glass of water

Full-strength concentrated extract: 15 drops in a glass of water

Oral spray: 3 sprayings

Evening Protocol: Walnut

At bedtime, take the recommended dose of one of the following forms of walnut extract.

D1 homeopathic strength: 100 drops in a glass of water
Full-strength concentrated extract: 15 drops in a glass of water
Oral spray: 3 sprayings

Spasmodic Colitis

Morning Protocol: Lingonberry

After rising in the morning, take the recommended dose of one of the following forms of lingonberry extract.

D1 homeopathic strength: 100 drops in a glass of water
Full-strength concentrated extract: 10 drops in a glass of water
Oral spray: 2 sprayings

Evening Protocol: Silver Linden

At bedtime, take the recommended dose of one of the following forms of silver linden extract.

D1 homeopathic strength: 150 drops in a glass of water
Full-strength concentrated extract: 15 drops in a glass of water
Oral spray: 3 sprayings

🍃 The Urinary System

The urinary system is comprised of the kidneys, which rid the blood of wastes by forming urine that it then sends into the bladder via the ureter tubes. It then passes through the urethra as it is eliminated from the body.

Thanks to its detoxifying qualities and diuretic action, gemmotherapy is very effective for treating the urinary system. Macerations of birch, juniper, lingonberry, and heather help to restore kidney function and can also be used in the treatment of kidney stones, bladder stones, and cystitis.

Kidney Failure

Morning Protocol: Juniper

After rising in the morning, take the recommended dose of one of the following forms of juniper extract.

D1 homeopathic strength: 50 drops in a glass of water
Full-strength concentrated extract: 10 drops in a glass of water
Oral spray: 3 sprayings

Evening Protocol: Birch

At bedtime, take the recommended dose of one of the following forms of birch extract.

D1 homeopathic strength: 50 drops in a glass of water
Full-strength concentrated extract: 15 drops in a glass of water
Oral spray: 3 sprayings

Kidney Stones

A combination of birch and heather is essential here and offers excellent results.

Morning and Evening Protocol: Birch and Heather

After rising in the morning and again at bedtime, take the recommended dose of one of the following forms of birch and heather extracts combined.

> *D1 homeopathic strength:* 100 drops of each in a glass of water
>
> *Full-strength concentrated extract:* 15 drops of each in a glass of water
>
> *Oral spray:* 2 sprayings of each

Cystitis

Morning Protocol: Lingonberry

After rising in the morning, take the recommended dose of one of the following forms of lingonberry extract.

> *D1 homeopathic strength:* 100 drops in a glass of water
>
> *Full-strength concentrated extract:* 15 drops in a glass of water
>
> *Oral spray:* 2 sprayings

Evening Protocol: Heather

At bedtime, take the recommended dose of one of the following forms of lingonberry extract.

> *D1 homeopathic strength:* 100 drops in a glass of water
>
> *Full-strength concentrated extract:* 15 drops in a glass of water
>
> *Oral spray:* 3 sprayings

❧ The Osteoarticular System

Our bones form a rigid framework for our bodies and protect our internal organs, as do the muscles, tendons, and ligaments that connect the bones to one another.

Gemmotherapy extracts are a leading choice in the selection of remedies for disorders affecting this system, due to both their effectiveness and the absence of any side effects. Unlike some pharmaceutical formulations, the buds used in gemmotherapy have a revitalizing action and bring about a regeneration throughout the body that can retard aging of the joints.

The macerations recommended here are from the buds or young shoots of pine, grapevine, and black currant, because of their anti-inflammatory action. Pine is effective on cartilage, grapevine works well in treating deformed joints, and black currant is generally effective for inflammation, which is often a key symptom of joint disorders.

Osteoporosis, another common disorder of the osteoarticular system, often occurs in women following menopause. Blackberry, sequoia, and grapevine all help to restore the body's mineral content and are very helpful in treating this disease.

Osteoarthritis in Individuals Younger than Age Sixty

Morning Protocol: Black Currant and Pine
After rising in the morning, take the recommended dose of one of the following forms of black currant and pine extracts.

D1 homeopathic strength: 150 drops of black currant extract and 50 drops of pine in a glass of water

Full-strength concentrated extract: 15 drops black currant and 10 drops pine in a glass of water

Oral spray: 3 sprayings black currant and 2 sprayings pine

Evening Protocol: Grapevine
At bedtime, take the recommended dose of one of the following forms of grapevine extract.

D1 homeopathic strength: 150 drops in a glass of water
Full-strength concentrated extract: 15 drops in a glass of water
Oral spray: 3 sprayings

Osteoarthritis in Individuals Older than Age Sixty

Depending on the individual case and gemmotherapy extract selected, treatment calls for the same three extracts as above, except that pine is replaced by sequoia to take advantage of its revitalizing properties.

Morning Protocol: Black Currant and Sequoia

After rising in the morning, take the recommended dose of one of the following forms of black currant and sequoia extracts.

D1 homeopathic strength: 50 drops of each in a glass of water
Full-strength concentrated extract: 15 drops of each in a glass of water
Oral spray: 3 sprayings of each

Evening Protocol: Grapevine

At bedtime, take the recommended dose of one of the following forms of grapevine extract.

D1 homeopathic strength: 150 drops in a glass of water
Full-strength concentrated extract: 15 drops in a glass of water
Oral spray: 3 sprayings

Osteoporosis—Decalcification

Morning Protocol: Sequoia and Blackberry

After rising in the morning, take the recommended dose of one of the following forms of sequoia and blackberry extracts.

D1 homeopathic strength: 50 drops of each in a glass of water
Full-strength concentrated extract: 15 drops of each in a glass of water
Oral spray: 3 sprayings of each

Evening Protocol: Grapevine

At bedtime, take the recommended dose of one of the following forms of grapevine extract.

D1 homeopathic strength: 100 drops in a glass of water

Full-strength concentrated extract: 10 drops in a glass of water

Oral spray: 2 sprayings

✤ The Skin

The most widespread organ of the body is the skin; it protects our bodies, forming the boundary to our insides.

Its function is also the elimination of wastes through perspiration and the maintenance of proper body temperature. It is resistant enough to protect our interior organs, while at the same time sensitive enough to the outside world to receive sensory messages.

This is why skin, an organ that serves protective, sensory, and eliminative functions simultaneously, is the most visible reflection of the state of a person's health. It is also a reflection of the nervous system, because it originates from the same embryonic tissue that gave birth to this system during gestation; and has a connection with the digestive tract and kidneys.

There are four essential gemmotherapy extracts for handling all dermatology issues: cedar, elm, walnut, and black currant.

Cedar is an excellent remedy for treating dry eczema and pruritus (itching) that has no apparent cause, elm is helpful against oozing and inflamed eczema, walnut helps infectious eczema, and black currant is valuable against all skin conditions of this nature because of it anti-inflammatory and anti-infectious properties.

Hives, which is an illness of allergenic origin often connected with the liver, can be treated with black currant, juniper, and alder.

Dry Eczema

Morning Protocol: Black Currant

After rising in the morning, take the recommended dose of one of the following forms of black currant extract.

D1 homeopathic strength: 150 drops in a glass of water
Full-strength concentrated extract: 15 drops in a glass of water
Oral spray: 3 sprayings

Evening Protocol: Elm

At bedtime, take the recommended dose of one of the following forms of elm extract.

> *D1 homeopathic strength:* 150 drops in a glass of water
> *Full-strength concentrated extract:* 15 drops in a glass of water
> *Oral spray:* 3 sprayings

Oozing Eczema

Morning Protocol: Black Currant

After rising in the morning, take the recommended dose of one of the following forms of black currant extract.

> *D1 homeopathic strength:* 150 drops in a glass of water
> *Full-strength concentrated extract:* 15 drops in a glass of water
> *Oral spray:* 3 sprayings

Evening Protocol: Walnut

At bedtime, take the recommended dose of one of the following forms of walnut extract.

> *D1 homeopathic strength:* 100 drops in a glass of water
> *Full-strength concentrated extract:* 10 drops in a glass of water
> *Oral spray:* 3 sprayings

Hives

Morning Protocol: Black Currant

After rising in the morning, take the recommended dose of one of the following forms of black currant extract.

> *D1 homeopathic strength:* 150 drops in a glass of water
> *Full-strength concentrated extract:* 15 drops in a glass of water
> *Oral spray:* 3 sprayings

Evening Protocol: Alder

At bedtime, take the recommended dose of one of the following forms of alder extract.

D1 homeopathic strength: 150 drops in a glass of water

Full-strength concentrated extract: 15 drops in a glass of water

Oral spray: 3 sprayings

&q The Endocrine System

Gemmotherapy has revealed some truly astonishing results in treatment of the endocrine system. In fact, it has been shown that the buds are able to regulate the quantity of essential hormones released by the body. This ability to increase or decrease hormones makes the macerations highly effective for illnesses that afflict the thyroid, adrenal glands, and male and female genital systems.

- *Action upon the thyroid.* Because there is often a connection between an overactive thyroid and a nervous system disorder, there are three bud extracts that can be quite helpful in the case of hyperthyroid: silver linden, fig, and wayfaring tree. Moreover, as hyperthyroidism is often responsible for causing disorders in the cardiac system, hawthorn can be useful.

  In the case of hypothyroid (underactive), the thyroid is functioning at a slowed pace that is not sufficient to produce the amount of thyroid hormones the body needs. Birch bud extract can delay the transition from this disorder to a more radical one in which a therapy of substitution is mandated, one in which thyroid extracts need to be taken to make up for what the body is not producing. The drawback to substitution therapies is that the body will cease production of hormones and other necessary chemicals if they are supplied externally.

- *Action on the adrenal glands.* Since the adrenal glands supply energy to the body and bolster its immune system, taking black currant extract will stimulate the body's defenses. Combining sequoia and oak with black currant will really boost this energizing action.

- *Gynecological action.* Raspberry buds have a proven effectiveness for dealing with menstrual cramps, no matter in which point of the cycle they occur, and can be combined with black currant extract for its anti-inflammatory properties. Menopause issues can be treated by raspberry extract in combination with rowan, lingonberry, and fig.

- *Action on the male reproductive system.* The slowing that occurs in male sexual function—or andropause—does not only affect erection and the nature of male sexual pleasure, but can also be visible in the domain of general behavior (fatigue, weight gain, lowered libido, erratic pains, prostate problems, and even depression). These conditions can be greatly alleviated by sequoia, oak (which stimulates testosterone), rosemary, and fig.

Hyperthyroid

Depending on the individual case, hawthorn, silver linden, fig, and wayfaring tree may be used to treat hyperthyroidism.

Morning Protocol: Wayfaring Tree and Hawthorn

After rising in the morning, take the recommended dose of one of the following forms of wayfaring tree and hawthorn extracts combined.

> *D1 homeopathic strength:* 50 drops wayfaring tree and 30 drops hawthorn in a glass of water
>
> *Full-strength concentrated extract:* 15 drops wayfaring tree and 10 drops hawthorn in a glass of water
>
> *Oral spray:* 3 sprayings of each

Evening Protocol: Silver Linden and Fig

At bedtime, take the recommended dose of one of the following forms of silver linden and fig extracts combined.

> *D1 homeopathic strength:* 100 drops each in a glass of water
>
> *Full-strength concentrated extract:* 15 drops each in a glass of water
>
> *Oral spray:* 2 sprayings of each

Hypothyroid

Morning and Evening Protocol: Birch

After rising in the morning and again before bedtime, take the recommended dose of one of the following forms of birch extract:

D1 homeopathic strength: 100 drops in a glass of water

Full-strength concentrated extract: 15 drops in a glass of water

Oral spray: 3 sprayings

Adrenal Gland Issues

Morning Protocol: Black Currant, Sequoia, and Oak

After rising in the morning, take the recommended dose of one of the following forms of black currant, sequoia, and oak extracts combined.

D1 homeopathic strength: 100 drops each in a glass of water

Full-strength concentrated extract: 15 drops each in a glass of water

Oral spray: 3 sprayings of each

Evening Protocol: Oak

At bedtime, take the recommended dose of one of the following forms of oak extract.

D1 homeopathic strength: 100 drops in a glass of water

Full-strength concentrated extract: 15 drops in a glass of water

Oral spray: 3 sprayings

Menstrual Problems

Morning and Evening Protocol: Raspberry and Black Currant

After rising in the morning and again before bedtime, take the recommended dose of one of the following forms of raspberry and black currant extracts combined.

D1 homeopathic strength: 50 drops each combined in a glass of water

Full-strength concentrated extract: 15 drops each combined in a glass of water

Oral spray: 3 sprayings of each

Menopause (Hot Flashes)

Depending on the individual case, raspberry, rowan, lingonberry, and fig may be used in treatment of the symptoms of menopause.

Morning and Evening Protocol: Raspberry, Rowan, Lingonberry, Fig

After rising in the morning and again before bedtime, take the recommended dose of one of the following forms of raspberry, rowan, lingonberry, and fig extracts combined.

D1 homeopathic strength: 50 drops each combined in a glass of water

Full-strength concentrated extract: 15 drops each combined in a glass of water

Oral spray: 3 sprayings of each

Male Problems

Depending on the individual case, sequoia, oak, rosemary, and fig may be used in treating the symptoms of male problems.

Morning and Evening Protocol: Sequoia, Oak, Rosemary, and Fig

After rising in the morning and again before bedtime, take the recommended dose of one of the following forms of sequoia, oak, rosemary, and fig extracts combined.

D1 homeopathic strength: 50 drops each combined in a glass of water

Full-strength concentrated extract: 15 drops each combined in a glass of water

Oral spray: 1 spraying of each

❧ Immune System—Allergies

The principle behind the appearance of an allergic reaction is quite simple. Our bodies are born with an immune system that developed over the course of our evolution to defend against foreign invaders (bacterium, fungi, and so on) and internal disruption (for example, cancers). Whenever the body senses that it is under attack, either internally or externally, it manufactures antibodies to defend itself. But sometimes too many of these antibodies are created and become aggressive irritants that then trigger the release of excessive amounts of histamine, a substance that causes allergic reactions.

Traditionally it was thought that heredity played the most important role in who was afflicted with allergies, but more recently other factors have come into play. Allergies have become problematic for a growing number of people because of the hostile nature of our polluted environment and the mental and emotional burden that stress puts on our bodies. This disorder, which puts the body on a hyper state of alert and overreaction, is particularly susceptible to treatment by gemmotherapy extracts. Macerations of embryonic plant matter have proven their effectiveness on allergies affecting the respiratory system (spasmodic coryza, hay fever, bronchial asthma), the skin (hives, eczema), the intestines (diarrhea, constipation), and the circulatory system (high blood pressure, migraines).

Gemmotherapy can provide valuable aid for regulating this situation with four particular extracts:

- *Black currant,* for its cortisone-like qualities
- *Rosemary,* for its hepatic action, as the liver plays a role in all allergies
- *Birch,* for its cleansing and purifying action and its regulating effect on the pituitary gland
- *Fig,* for its psychosomatic action

Recommended Treatment for All Allergy Symptoms

Depending on the individual case, black currant, rosemary, birch, and fig may be useful for allergies.

Morning and Evening Protocol

After rising in the morning and again before bedtime, take the recommended dose of one of the following forms of black currant, rosemary, birch, and fig extracts combined.

D1 homeopathic strength: 50 drops each combined in a glass of water

Full-strength concentrated extract: 15 drops each combined in a glass of water

Oral spray: 2 sprayings of each

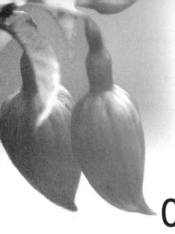

Conclusion

As we have seen, gemmotherapy is one of the most exciting therapeutic innovations to appear in recent years in holistic medicine, and undoubtedly will continue to grow and enrich the fields of homeopathy and herbal medicine. It helps remind us that despite major product developments in the pharmaceutical industry, we can still derive great benefit from the invaluable services plants are able to offer.

The scientific world has a tendency to neglect and scoff at this plant world, and in the name of progress, we've already lost many species of plants that we can never regain. Because of thoughtless mass harvesting, the destruction of plant habitat, and the ravages caused by pollution, humanity stands on the brink of extinction. We are at a point where only a wager of double or nothing may determine whether we live or disappear from the face of the earth.

It is important to raise our level of awareness. We already have everything we need to lead fulfilling and happy lives; all the necessary elements are right around us, and we are part of them. The mineral world forms our bones, the plant world works with our blood, and the animal world provides a template for our organs. We should respect all of them and learn how to make use of the help they offer. The new branch of medical learning, gemmotherapy, falls squarely into this perspective.

❧ Resources

At this time, full-strength concentrated extracts are not available for purchase in retail markets but are available to doctors who can order the remedies for their patients. However, D1 homeopathic-strength remedies are available for purchase by the general public and are becoming increasingly available in retail markets. The following companies offer a variety of products, including D1 homeopathic-strength dilutions and full-strength concentrated extracts.

Boiron
6 Campus Boulevard
Newtown Square, PA 19073-3267
(800) BOIRON-1
www.boironusa.com
Sells D1 homeopathic-strength remedies

Gemmos
550 Grand St.
Brooklyn, NY 11211
Phone: (877) 417-6298
Fax: (718) 599-1997
www.gemmos-usa.com
Sells HerbalGem full-strength concentrates and D1 homeopathic-strength remedies; mainly a wholesaler, but a very informative website

HerbalGem
Bihain, 28
Vielsalm, B 6690
Belgium
Phone: 32 (0)80 418 154
Fax: 32 (0)80 418 153
www.herbalgem.com
Founded by Philippe Andrianne, sells only full-strength extracts

Organic Pharmacy
3 Tingle Alley, Ste E.
Asheville, NC 28801-2948
Phone: (800) 819-6742
Fax: (828) 225-8859
www.organicpharmacy.org
Sells D1 homeopathic-strength remedies by Boiron and Dynamic Nutritional Associates

PSC Plant Stem Cell Nutrition
37 Front Street, 2nd Floor
Greenport, NY 11944
Phone: (631) 477-6696
Fax: (631) 477-6695
www.plantstemcells.net
Sells full-strength extracts by PSC and Forza Vitale

Rockwell Nutrition
www.rockwellnutrition.com
Prefers to be contacted via e-mail/no phone provided. Sells D1 homeopathic-strength remedies by Juglans, Unda, and Seroyal

SPREMA Gemmotherapy, Ltd.
1 Albion Terrace
Box Hill, Corsham
Wiltshire SN13 8HR
United Kingdom
Phone: 44 1225 742 223
www.gemmotherapy.com
Founded by Nick Churchill, a gemmotherapy pioneer. Sells DH1 potentized remedies in protective violet glass bottles and will be offering concentrates by late 2010. Churchill reports, "We could produce sprays if required."

Index